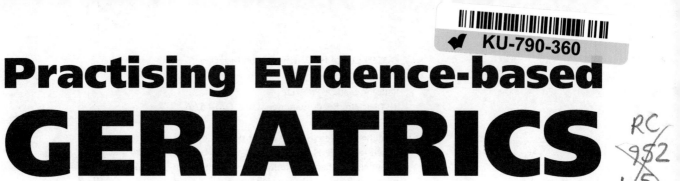

Practising Evidence-based
GERIATRICS

Sharon E Straus

David L Sackett

At the NHS R&D Centre for Evidence-based Medicine
Nuffield Department of Clinical Medicine
Level 5, John Radcliffe Hospital
Headley Way, Headington
Oxford OX3 9DU

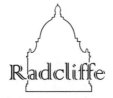

Radcliffe Medical Press
18 Marcham Road, Abingdon, Oxon OX14 1AA, UK
Tel: 01235 528820 Fax: 01235 528830
e-mail: medical@radpress.win-uk.net

© 1999 Centre for Evidence-based Medicine

Radcliffe Medical Press Ltd
18 Marcham Road, Abingdon, Oxon OX14 1AA

British Library Cataloguing in Publication Data

A catalogue record for this book is available from the British Library.

ISBN 1 85775 394 1

Typeset by Advance Typesetting Ltd, Oxfordshire
Printed and bound by Hobbs the Printers, Totton, Hampshire

SESSION	TOPIC

CONTENTS

ACKNOWLEDGEMENTS

Radcliffe Medical Press acknowledges with gratitude the kind permission granted by publishers of the citation references for the full papers to be reproduced at the beginning of each session. These permissions prohibit further reproduction by photocopying or by electronic means and if this facility is required, further permission should be obtained from the source quoted in each case.

Extracts from *Evidence-based Medicine: how to practice and teach EBM* (David Sackett *et al.*) which appear at the back of this manual are reproduced with the kind permission of Harcourt Brace & Co Ltd.

This is a syllabus for a 7 session course for clinicians with an interest in geriatric medicine on how to practice evidence-based medicine: that is, how to integrate our individual clinical expertise with a critical appraisal of the best available external clinical evidence from systematic research.

We see the practice of evidence-based medicine as a process of life-long, self-directed, problem-based learning in which caring for one's own patients creates the need for clinically important information about diagnosis, prognosis, therapy, and other clinical and healthcare issues, in which its practitioners:

1   convert these information needs into answerable questions;

2   track down, with maximum efficiency, the best evidence with which to answer them (making best use of the increasing variety of sources of primary and secondary evidence);

3   critically appraise that evidence for its validity (closeness to the truth), importance (size of effect) and usefulness (clinical applicability);

4   integrate the appraisal with clinical expertise and apply the results in clinical practice; and

5   evaluate their own performance.

This syllabus is designed to help clinicians develop and improve those skills. In addition, it is designed to help Membership candidates prepare for the EBM portions of the Membership Examination.

Each of its 7 sessions is divided into 2 parts:

Part A: Going through the 5 steps with a patient, focusing on step 3 (critical appraisal), step 4 (integration with clinical expertise), and step 5 (self-evaluation).

Part B: Skills training, focusing on step 1 (forming answerable clinical questions) and step 2 (finding the best evidence), in which we introduce a variety of sources of evidence plus some strategies for analysing, summarising and storing the evidence in the form of one-page summaries ("Critically Appraised Topics" or CATs).

Evidence-based Medicine: what it is and what it isn't

This is the text of an editorial from the *British Medical Journal* on 13th January 1996
(*BMJ* 1996; **312**: 71–2)

Authors:

David L Sackett, Professor, NHS Research and Development Centre for Evidence-based Medicine, Oxford.

William MC Rosenberg, Clinical Tutor in Medicine, Nuffield Department of Clinical Medicine, Oxford.

JA Muir Gray, Director of Research and Development, Anglia and Oxford Regional Health Authority, Milton Keynes.

R Brian Haynes, Professor of Medicine and Clinical Epidemiology, McMaster University Hamilton, Canada.

W Scott Richardson, Rochester, USA.

Evidence-based Medicine, whose philosophical origins extend back to mid-19th century Paris and earlier, remains a hot topic for clinicians, public health practitioners, purchasers, planners, and the public. There are now frequent workshops in how to practice and teach it (one sponsored by this journal will be held in London on April 24th); undergraduate [1] and post-graduate training programmes [2] are incorporating it [3] (or pondering how to do so); British centres for evidence-based practice have been established or planned in adult medicine, child health, surgery, pathology, pharmacotherapy, nursing, general practice, and dentistry; the Cochrane Collaboration and the York Centre for Review and Dissemination in York are providing systematic reviews of the effects of health care; new evidence-based practice journals are being launched; and it has become a common topic in the lay media. But enthusiasm has been mixed with some negative reaction [4–6]. Criticism has ranged from evidence-based medicine being old-hat to it being a dangerous innovation, perpetrated by the arrogant to serve cost-cutters and suppress clinical freedom. As evidence-based medicine continues to evolve and adapt, now is a useful time to refine the discussion of what it is and what it is not.

Evidence-based medicine is the conscientious, explicit and judicious use of current best evidence in making decisions about the care of individual patients. The practice of evidence-based medicine means integrating individual clinical expertise with the best available external clinical evidence from systematic research. By individual clinical expertise we mean the proficiency and judgement that individual clinicians acquire through clinical experience and clinical practice. Increased expertise is reflected in many ways, but especially in more effective and efficient diagnosis and in the more thoughtful identification and compassionate use of individual patients' predicaments, rights, and preferences in making clinical decisions about their care. By best available external clinical evidence we mean clinically relevant research, often from the basic sciences of medicine, but especially from patient centred clinical research into the accuracy and precision of diagnostic tests (including the clinical examination), the power of prognostic markers, and the efficacy and safety of therapeutic, rehabilitative, and preventive regimens. External clinical evidence both invalidates previously accepted diagnostic tests and treatments and replaces them with new ones that are more powerful, more accurate, more efficacious, and safer.

Good doctors use both individual clinical expertise and the best available external evidence, and neither alone is enough. Without clinical expertise, practice risks becoming tyrannised by evidence, for even excellent external evidence may be inapplicable to or inappropriate for an individual patient. Without current best evidence, practice risks becoming rapidly out of date, to the detriment of patients.

This description of what evidence-based medicine is helps clarify what evidence-based medicine is not. Evidence-based medicine is neither old-hat nor impossible to practice. The argument that everyone already is doing it falls before evidence of striking variations in both the integration of patient values into our clinical behaviour [7] and in the rates with which clinicians provide interventions to their patients [8]. The difficulties that clinicians face in keeping abreast of all the medical advances reported in primary journals are obvious from a comparison of the time required for reading (for general medicine, enough to examine

Introduction

19 articles per day, 365 days per year [9]) with the time available (well under an hour per week by British medical consultants, even on self-reports [10]).

The argument that evidence-based medicine can be conducted only from ivory towers and armchairs is refuted by audits in the front lines of clinical care where at least some inpatient clinical teams in general medicine [11], psychiatry (JR Geddes, et al, Royal College of Psychiatrists winter meeting, January 1996), and surgery (P McCulloch, personal communication) have provided evidence-based care to the vast majority of their patients. Such studies show that busy clinicians who devote their scarce reading time to selective, efficient, patient-driven searching, appraisal and incorporation of the best available evidence can practice evidence-based medicine.

Evidence-based medicine is not "cook-book" medicine. Because it requires a bottom-up approach that integrates the best external evidence with individual clinical expertise and patient-choice, it cannot result in slavish, cook-book approaches to individual patient care. External clinical evidence can inform, but can never replace, individual clinical expertise, and it is this expertise that decides whether the external evidence applies to the individual patient at all and, if so, how it should be integrated into a clinical decision. Similarly, any external guideline must be integrated with individual clinical expertise in deciding whether and how it matches the patient's clinical state, predicament, and preferences, and thus whether it should be applied. Clinicians who fear top-down cook-books will find the advocates of evidence-based medicine joining them at the barricades.

Evidence-based medicine is not cost-cutting medicine. Some fear that evidence-based medicine will be hijacked by purchasers and managers to cut the costs of health care. This would not only be a misuse of evidence-based medicine but suggests a fundamental misunderstanding of its financial consequences. Doctors practising evidence-based medicine will identify and apply the most efficacious interventions to maximise the quality and quantity of life for individual patients; this may raise rather than lower the cost of their care.

Evidence-based medicine is not restricted to randomised trials and meta-analyses. It involves tracking down the best external evidence with which to answer our clinical questions. To find out about the accuracy of a diagnostic test, we need to find proper cross-sectional studies of patients clinically suspected of harbouring the relevant disorder, not a randomised trial. For a question about prognosis, we need proper follow-up studies of patients assembled at a uniform, early point in the clinical course of their disease. And sometimes the evidence we need will come from the basic sciences such as genetics or immunology. It is when asking questions about therapy that we should try to avoid the non-experimental approaches, since these routinely lead to false-positive conclusions about efficacy. Because the randomised trial, and especially the systematic review of several randomised trials, is so much more likely to inform us and so much less likely to mislead us, it has become the "gold standard" for judging whether a treatment does more good than harm. However, some questions about therapy do not require randomised trials (successful interventions for otherwise fatal conditions) or cannot wait for the trials to be conducted. And if no randomised trial has been carried out for our patient's predicament, we follow the trail to the next best external evidence and work from there.

Despite its ancient origins, evidence-based medicine remains a relatively young discipline whose positive impacts are just beginning to be validated [12, 13], and it will continue to evolve. This evolution will be enhanced as several undergraduate, post-graduate, and continuing medical education programmes adopt and adapt it to their learners' needs. These programmes, and their evaluation, will provide further information and understanding about what evidence-based medicine is, and what it is not.

References

1   British Medical Association: *Report of the working party on medical education*. London: British Medical Association, 1995.

2   Standing Committee on Postgraduate Medical and Dental Education: *Creating a better learning environment in hospitals: 1 Teaching hospital doctors and dentists to teach*. London: SCOPME, 1994.

3   General Medical Council: *Education Committee Report*. London: General Medical Council, 1994.

4   Grahame-Smith D: Evidence-based medicine: Socratic dissent. *BMJ* 1995; 310: 1126-7.

5   Evidence-based medicine, in its place (editorial). *Lancet* 1995; 346: 785.

6   Correspondence. Evidence-based Medicine. *Lancet* 1995; 346: 1171–2.

7   Weatherall DJ: The inhumanity of medicine. *BMJ* 1994; 308: 1671–2.

8   House of Commons Health Committee. *Priority setting in the NHS: purchasing*. First report sessions 1994–95. London: HMSO, 1995, (HC 134–1.)

9   Davidoff F, Haynes B, Sackett D, Smith R: Evidence-based medicine; a new journal to help doctors identify the information they need. *BMJ* 1995; 310: 1085–6.

10 Sackett DL: Surveys of self-reported reading times of consultants in Oxford, Birmingham, Milton-Keynes, Bristol, Leicester, and Glasgow, 1995. In Rosenberg WMC, Richardson WS, Haynes RB, Sackett DL. *Evidence-based Medicine*. London: Churchill-Livingstone, 1999.

11 Ellis J, Mulligan I, Rowe J, Sackett DL: Inpatient general medicine is evidence based. *Lancet* 1995; 346: 407–10.

12 Bennett RJ, Sackett DL, Haynes RB, Neufeld VR: A controlled trial of teaching critical appraisal of the clinical literature to medical students. *JAMA* 1987; 257: 2451–4.

13 Shin JH, Haynes RB, Johnston ME: Effect of problem-based, self-directed undergraduate education on life-long learning. *Can Med Assoc J* 1993; 148: 969–76.

PART A

Critical appraisal of a clinical article about therapy

You see a 75-year old patient referred to you by his GP because of raised blood pressure. His past medical history is remarkable for mild asthma but he is otherwise well. His GP has enclosed a note stating that the patient's blood pressure has been 160–190/80–90 for the past three months. The patient's wife is on an ACE-I and has had no adverse effects and the patient wondered if he could take it as well. You explain to the patient that evidence from trials suggest that diuretics and beta blockers should be used as the initial treatment strategy because they are known to decrease the risk of stroke. The patient asks to look at this evidence with you. You formulate the question: 'In patients with isolated systolic hypertension, do diuretics decrease the risk of stroke and death?'

You start up *Best Evidence,* enter 'hypertension' and 'stroke' and you find the abstract and commentary for the randomised controlled trial assessing the prevention of stroke with antihypertensive therapy. The abstract and commentary look helpful so you decide to go to the library and copy the original article: *JAMA* (1991) **265:** 3255–64. You make a follow-up appointment with your patient and tell him that you will discuss the evidence with him at that time.

Read the article and decide:
1 Is the evidence from this randomised trial valid?
2 If valid, is this evidence important?
3 If valid and important, can you apply this evidence in caring for your patient?

If you want to read some strategies for answering these sorts of questions, you could have a look at pp 91–6, 133–41 and 166–72 in *Evidence-based Medicine.*

PART B

Asking answerable clinical questions

1 We illustrate the importance, strategies and tactics of formulating clinical questions and work with you on the three to four parts of the question.

2 Participants break up into groups of two, discuss patients they cared for in the previous week, and generate questions they think are important concerning their patients' therapy, diagnosis and prognosis.

3 In larger groups, we review and refine the questions, and then keep track of them as possible questions to use in later sessions devoted to searching for the best evidence.

Original Contributions

Prevention of Stroke by Antihypertensive Drug Treatment in Older Persons With Isolated Systolic Hypertension

Final Results of the Systolic Hypertension in the Elderly Program (SHEP)

SHEP Cooperative Research Group

Objective.—To assess the ability of antihypertensive drug treatment to reduce the risk of nonfatal and fatal (total) stroke in isolated systolic hypertension.

Design.—Multicenter, randomized, double-blind, placebo-controlled.

Setting.—Community-based ambulatory population in tertiary care centers.

Participants.—4736 persons (1.06%) from 447 921 screenees aged 60 years and above were randomized (2365 to active treatment, 2371 to placebo). Systolic blood pressure ranged from 160 to 219 mm Hg and diastolic blood pressure was less than 90 mm Hg. Of the participants, 3161 were not receiving antihypertensive medication at initial contact, and 1575 were. The average systolic blood pressure was 170 mm Hg; average diastolic blood pressure, 77 mm Hg. The mean age was 72 years, 57% were women, and 14% were black.

Interventions.—Participants were stratified by clinical center and by antihypertensive medication status at initial contact. For step 1 of the trial, dose 1 was chlorthalidone, 12.5 mg/d, or matching placebo; dose 2 was 25 mg/d. For step 2, dose 1 was atenolol, 25 mg/d, or matching placebo; dose 2 was 50 mg/d.

Main Outcome Measures.—*Primary.*—Nonfatal and fatal (total) stroke. *Secondary.*—Cardiovascular and coronary morbidity and mortality, all-cause mortality, and quality of life measures.

Results.—Average follow-up was 4.5 years. The 5-year average systolic blood pressure was 155 mm Hg for the placebo group and 143 mm Hg for the active treatment group, and the 5-year average diastolic blood pressure was 72 and 68 mm Hg, respectively. The 5-year incidence of total stroke was 5.2 per 100 participants for active treatment and 8.2 per 100 for placebo. The relative risk by proportional hazards regression analysis was 0.64 (*P* = .0003). For the secondary end point of clinical nonfatal myocardial infarction plus coronary death, the relative risk was 0.73. Major cardiovascular events were reduced (relative risk, 0.68). For deaths from all causes, the relative risk was 0.87.

Conclusion.—In persons aged 60 years and over with isolated systolic hypertension, antihypertensive stepped-care drug treatment with low-dose chlorthalidone as step 1 medication reduced the incidence of total stroke by 36%, with 5-year absolute benefit of 30 events per 1000 participants. Major cardiovascular events were reduced, with 5-year absolute benefit of 55 events per 1000.

(JAMA. 1991;265:3255-3264)

THIS article presents the final results of the Systolic Hypertension in the Elderly Program (SHEP), a double-blind, randomized, placebo-controlled trial of treatment for isolated systolic hypertension (ISH) in persons 60 years of age and older. The full-scale SHEP study, begun in 1984, set as its primary objective "the determination of whether antihypertensive drug treatment reduces risk of total stroke (nonfatal and fatal) in

See the end of the article for a list of the principal investigators of the Systolic Hypertension in the Elderly Program.

Reprint requests to Clinical Trials Branch, Division of Epidemiology and Clinical Applications, National Heart, Lung, and Blood Institute, Federal Building, Room 5C-10B, 7550 Wisconsin Ave, Bethesda, MD 20892 (Dr Jeffrey L. Probstfield).

a multi-ethnic cohort of men and women age 60 years and older with ISH."[1] Previous trials have demonstrated beneficial effects of antihypertensive treatment of diastolic hypertension on major morbidity and mortality, but none has investigated the ability to influence these events for persons with ISH.[2-21]

For editorial comment see p 3301.

Isolated systolic hypertension is increasingly prevalent with age, especially in those aged 60 years and above. Epidemiologic studies have demonstrated an increase in risk of stroke, other cardiovascular diseases, and death for those with ISH, independent of other risk factors.[22-28]

The SHEP pilot study demonstrated the feasibility of undertaking trials in older people with ISH, including ability to recruit participants. It also established ability of drug therapy to reduce blood pressure among persons with ISH.[29] For SHEP, ISH was defined as systolic blood pressure (SBP) greater than 160 mm Hg and diastolic blood pressure (DBP) less than 90 mm Hg, based on the average of four measurements at two baseline visits.[1,30]

Secondary objectives included assessment of the relationship of antihypertensive treatment to (1) multiple cardiovascular morbidity and mortality end points, including cardiac end points; (2) cause-specific and all-cause mortality; (3) multi-infarct dementia, clinical depression, and deterioration of cognitive function; (4) possible adverse effects; (5) hospitalizations and intermediate or skilled nursing facility admissions; (6) falls and fractures; and (7) multiple indexes of quality of life.[1,30]

The SHEP protocol also stipulated two other questions for investigation as subgroup hypotheses[1]: (1) Would treatment of ISH reduce the frequency of total stroke (fatal and nonfatal) similarly in those receiving and not receiving antihypertensive medication at initial contact? (2) Would treatment of ISH reduce the incidence of sudden cardiac death or of coronary death plus nonfatal myocardial infarction similarly in those free of baseline electrocardiographic (ECG) abnormalities and in those with such abnormalities?

METHODS

The design and methods of SHEP have been reported in detail elsewhere.[1,30,31] They are summarized here.

Sample Size

The SHEP design specified a sample size of 4800 participants to test the primary hypothesis.[32] This sample size was used to detect a difference of at least 32% in total stroke incidence with 90% power and a two-sided α of .05.

Recruitment and Screening

For recruitment, SHEP used primarily mass mailing and community screening techniques.[33] All identified potential participants underwent an initial contact to exclude individuals ineligible by age, blood pressure, and other criteria.[31] One seated blood pressure reading was taken. All blood pressures during screening and trial follow-up were measured by trained, certified technicians using standardized techniques with a Hawksley random-zero manometer.[34] The SBP was defined as the reading at the first Korotkoff sound and DBP as the reading at the last Korotkoff sound. For persons not receiving antihypertensive drugs who had a first SBP reading greater than 150 mm Hg, two more readings were taken. When the mean of the last two readings was between 160 and 219 mm Hg for SBP and less than 100 mm Hg for DBP, the person was eligible for the first baseline visit.

Persons receiving antihypertensive medication at initial contact who had SBPs between 130 and 219 mm Hg and DBPs less than 85 mm Hg and who were free of major illness were eligible for a drug withdrawal procedure. They were asked to obtain permission from their personal physicians and to sign an informed consent form for drug withdrawal. They were then monitored at multiple drug evaluation visits during a 2- to 8-week period to determine blood pressure eligibility off medication.

The baseline phase consisted of two visits. Eligibility was determined based on study inclusion and exclusion criteria. When the average of four seated blood pressure measurements, two at each of these visits, was between 160 and 219 mm Hg for SBP and less than 90

mm Hg for DBP, the participant was eligible for the trial. Persons were excluded on the basis of history and/or signs of specified major cardiovascular diseases.[31] Other major diseases, eg, cancer, alcoholic liver disease, established renal dysfunction, with competing risk for the SHEP primary end point or the presence of medical management problems, were also exclusions. Screenees also underwent a physical examination, and a 12-lead ECG was done, with a 2-minute rhythm strip.

Those remaining eligible at the second baseline visit underwent behavioral assessment (including cognition, mood, and activities of daily living),[35] signed an additional informed consent form for participation in the trial, and had blood drawn.

Randomization

At the completion of the second baseline visit, after verification of eligibility, screenees were randomly allocated by the coordinating center to one of two treatment groups. Randomization was stratified by clinical center and by antihypertensive medication status at initial contact.

Treatment Program

Participants were randomized in a double-blind manner to a once-daily dose of either active drug treatment or matching placebo. Baseline SBP (average of four seated blood pressure readings at the first and second baseline visits) was used to establish a goal blood pressure for each participant. For individuals with SBPs greater than 180 mm Hg, the goal was a reduction to less than 160 mm Hg. For those with SBPs between 160 and 179 mm Hg, the goal was a reduction of at least 20 mm Hg.

The objective of the stepped-care treatment program was to use the minimal amount of medication to maintain SBP at or below the goal. All participants were given chlorthalidone, 12.5 mg/d, or matching placebo (step 1 medication). Drug dosage was doubled (including matching placebo) for participants failing to achieve the SBP goal at follow-up visits. If the SBP goal was not reached at the maximal dose of step 1 medication, atenolol, 25 mg/d, or matching placebo was added as the usual step 2 drug. When atenolol was contraindicated, reserpine, 0.05 mg/d, or matching placebo could be substituted. When required to reach the blood pressure goal, the dosage of the step 2 drug could be doubled. Potassium supplements were given to all participants who had serum potassium concentrations below 3.5 mmol/L at two consecutive visits.

Follow-up Procedures

The SHEP participants were followed up monthly until SBP reached the goal or until the maximum level of stepped-care treatment was reached.[31] All participants had quarterly visits from the date of randomization, at which they underwent measurement of blood pressure (average of two readings), heart rate, and body weight, and a general medical history and detailed review of medication use (prescribed and over the counter) were done. At semiannual visits, standardized questionnaires were administered to screen for depression and dementia.[35,36] Annual visits also included (1) a detailed medical history, (2) a complete physical examination, (3) laboratory tests, and (4) behavioral assessment. An ECG was also done at the second and final annual visits. Other visits were scheduled when indicated, eg, SBP above the goal, SBP or DBP above the escape criteria (see below), low serum potassium concentration (<3.2 mmol/L), or as requested by the clinician or participant. Blood pressure above a priori escape criteria, despite maximal stepped-care therapy, was an indication for prescribing known active drug therapy. Escape criteria included SBP greater than 240 mm Hg at a single visit, DBP greater than 115 mm Hg at a single visit, sustained SBP greater than 220 mm Hg, or sustained DBP greater than 90 mm Hg.

When adverse conditions occurred that were considered drug related, the dosage of the study medication could be reduced, or therapy could be discontinued. Whenever the dosage was reduced or therapy was discontinued, consideration was given to resuming drug therapy when it appeared safe, when the participant's blood pressure was above the goal, and when the participant agreed.

Ascertainment of End Points

Total stroke was the primary end point. Stroke was defined as rapid onset of a new neurologic deficit attributed to obstruction or rupture in the arterial system.[37] The defined deficit had to persist for at least 24 hours unless death supervened and had to include specific localizing findings confirmed by neurologic examination or brain scan, with no evidence of an underlying nonvascular cause. Determination of fatal stroke was based on either autopsy or death certificate plus data on preterminal hospitalization with a definite diagnosis of stroke. Definitions of individual secondary end points were (1) sudden cardiac death—death within 1 hour of the onset of severe cardiac symptoms, unrelated

Prevention of Stroke—SHEP Cooperative Research Group

to other known causes; (2) rapid cardiac death—death within 1 to 24 hours of the onset of severe cardiac symptoms, unrelated to other known causes; (3) nonfatal myocardial infarction—typical symptoms consistent with acute myocardial infarction plus either typical ECG changes (including new Q waves) or significant enzyme elevation (1.25 times normal), but not including silent myocardial infarction; (4) fatal myocardial infarction—autopsy diagnosis or death certificate diagnosis plus preterminal hospitalization, with a definite or suspected diagnosis of myocardial infarction within 4 weeks of death; (5) left ventricular failure—a symptom, such as significant dyspnea, plus a chest roentgenogram characteristic of congestive heart failure, or an abnormal physical sign, such as rales or 2+ (moderate) ankle edema; (6) other cardiovascular death—presumed myocardial infarction that did not meet diagnostic criteria, or other cardiovascular causes; (7) transient ischemic attack—rapid onset of a focal neurologic deficit lasting more than 30 seconds and less than 24 hours, presumed to be due to cerebral ischemia, with no evidence of an underlying nonvascular cause; (8) coronary artery therapeutic procedures—coronary artery bypass graft or coronary angioplasty; and (9) renal dysfunction—serum creatinine concentration greater than 265.2 μmol/L. For combined end points, participants with multiple end points were counted only once.

Information related to study end points was collected by clinic staff. For suspected stroke and transient ischemic attack, a standardized neurological evaluation was carried out by a SHEP neurologist. For suspected stroke, this evaluation and notes by the attending neurologist and scans or other studies of the brain were forwarded to the coordinating center. For participants with suspected myocardial infarction or left ventricular failure, data requested included ECGs, cardiac enzymes, chest roentgenogram reports, and other clinical information. Death certificates and autopsy reports were obtained for decedents. For hospitalizations and nursing home admissions, discharge or admission sheets were obtained.

Occurrence of study events listed above was confirmed by a coding panel of three physicians blind to randomization allocation. For a neurological event, the coding panel included two neurologists. For myocardial infarction, left ventricular failure, and all causes of death, the panel included at least one cardiologist.

Possible adverse clinical and biochemical effects of the SHEP treat-

JAMA, June 26, 1991—Vol 265, No. 24

Table 1.—Baseline Characteristics of Randomized SHEP Participants by Treatment Group*

Characteristic	Active Treatment Group	Placebo Group	Total
No. randomized	2365	2371	**4736**
Age, y			
Average†	71.6 (6.7)	71.5 (6.7)	71.6 (6.7)
%			
60-69	41.1	41.8	41.5
70-79	44.9	44.7	44.8
≥80	14.0	13.4	13.7
Race-sex, %‡			
Black men	4.9	4.3	4.6
Black women	8.9	9.7	9.3
White men	38.8	38.4	38.6
White women	47.4	47.7	47.5
Education, y†	11.7 (3.5)	11.7 (3.4)	11.7 (3.5)
Blood pressure, mm Hg†			
Systolic	170.5 (9.5)	170.1 (9.2)	170.3 (9.4)
Diastolic	76.7 (9.6)	76.4 (9.8)	76.6 (9.7)
Antihypertensive medication at initial contact, %	33.0	33.5	33.3
Smoking, %			
Current smokers	12.6	12.9	12.7
Past smokers	36.6	37.6	37.1
Never smokers	50.8	49.6	50.2
Alcohol use, %			
Never	21.5	21.7	21.6
Formerly	9.6	10.4	10.0
Occasionally	55.2	53.9	54.5
Daily or nearly daily	13.7	14.0	13.8
History of myocardial infarction, %	4.9	4.9	4.9
History of stroke, %	1.5	1.3	1.4
History of diabetes, %	10.0	10.2	10.1
Carotid bruits, %	6.4	7.9	7.1
Pulse rate, beats/min†§	70.3 (10.5)	71.3 (10.5)	70.8 (10.5)
Body-mass index, kg/m²†	27.5 (4.9)	27.5 (5.1)	27.5 (5.0)
Serum cholesterol, mmol/L†			
Total	6.1 (1.2)	6.1 (1.1)	6.1 (1.1)
High-density lipoprotein	1.4 (0.4)	1.4 (0.4)	1.4 (0.4)
Depressive symptoms, %‖	11.1	11.0	11.1
Evidence of cognitive impairment, %¶	0.3	0.5	0.4
No limitation of activities of daily living, %§	95.4	93.8	94.6
Baseline electrocardiographic abnormalities, %#	61.3	60.7	61.0

*SHEP indicates the Systolic Hypertension in the Elderly Program.
†Values are mean (SD).
‡Included among the whites were 204 Orientals (5% of whites), 84 Hispanics (2% of whites), and 41 classified as "other" (1% of whites).
§$P<.05$ for the active treatment group compared with the placebo group.
‖Depressive symptom scale score of 7 or greater.[31]
¶Cognitive impairment scale score of 4 or greater.[31]
#One or more of the following Minnesota codes: 1.1 to 1.3 (Q/QS), 3.1 to 3.4 (high R waves), 4.1 to 4.4 (ST depression), 5.1 to 5.4 (T wave changes), 6.1 to 6.8 (AV conduction defects), 7.1 to 7.8 (ventricular conduction defects), 8.1 to 8.6 (arrhythmias), and 9.1 to 9.3 and 9.5 (miscellaneous items).[50,51]

ments were evaluated by (1) using a standardized questionnaire that asked participants questions about side effects at annual visits, at visits after the administration of study drugs was started or stepped up, and at visits at which complaints were thought to be due to SHEP medication and by (2) examining serum chemistry data from annual laboratory evaluations.

The behavioral assessment included a questionnaire to detect depression and dementia, administered at baseline and semiannually. Based on specified questionnaire scores,[36] participants were referred for expert diagnostic evaluation[31] in accordance with American Psychiatric Association criteria.[38] A diagnosis of

dementia had to be confirmed by the SHEP coding panel, including two neurologists. A diagnosis of depression was not reviewed centrally.

Statistical Analyses

Comparability of baseline characteristics of the two treatment groups was ascertained by χ^2 tests for categorical variables and standard normal (z) tests for continuous variables. The primary hypothesis was assessed with the log-rank test[39] using time to first stroke as the variable of interest. Cumulative event rates were calculated using life table methods. Relative risks and percentage differences were calculated by proportional hazards regression analy-

Table 2.—Participants Receiving Antihypertensive Medication by Year of Follow-up

| | No. of Participants at End of Year* | | Medication Status, % | | | | | | | |
| | | | | Treated with Known Active Drug Only | | Untreated | | Unknown | |
Year	Active Treatment Group	Placebo Group	Treated (Active Treatment Group)	Active Treatment Group	Placebo Group	Active Treatment Group	Placebo Group	Active Treatment Group	Placebo Group
1	2342	2336	90.3	3.4	13.1	5.5	81.4	4.1	5.5
2	2308	2293	89.2	8.7	23.7	6.7	70.9	4.1	5.4
3	2241	2270	89.4	12.8	32.7	7.6	62.8	3.0	4.5
4	1605	1591	90.0	17.1	38.5	8.0	58.8	2.0	2.8
5	773	738	89.7	21.5	44.4	8.9	53.6	1.4	2.0

*The number of participants drops off in years 4 and 5 mainly due to follow-up time.

sis[40] using the entire duration of follow-up. All analyses were by treatment assignment at randomization. Two subgroup hypotheses were specified a priori. Subgroup hypotheses were tested by the proportional hazards model using the appropriate interaction term.[40] Power analyses for the subgroup hypotheses have been previously described.[1]

A Data and Safety Monitoring Board met twice per year to review unblinded data on efficacy and safety. The board used stochastic curtailment[41,42] to evaluate whether the trial should be stopped early. This was used to calculate the probability that a conclusion based on interim study results would remain unchanged at the trial's end, even if there were no benefit from antihypertensive treatment for the rest of the trial.

RESULTS

Recruitment

Recruitment was done at 16 clinical centers between March 1, 1985, and January 15, 1988. Details of recruitment results have been published elsewhere.[33] Altogether, 447 921 individuals aged 60 years and above were identified and contacted; 11.6% met initial criteria, and 2.7% completed baseline visit 1. Of those individuals, 64% were eligible for baseline visit 2; of those, 70% were eligible for randomization; of those, 88% were randomized.

Screenees meeting blood pressure criteria and not receiving antihypertensive medication proceeded directly through two baseline visits; 3161 such participants were randomized. Those taking medication (193 620 persons [43.2%]) and meeting blood pressure criteria underwent drug withdrawal as previously described; 1575 such participants were randomized. A total of 4736 participants were randomized into the trial, two thirds of whom were not receiving antihypertensive medication at initial contact. The yield from initial contact to randomization for those not

Table 3.—Mean Systolic and Diastolic Blood Pressures by Treatment Group and Year of Follow-up

| | Blood Pressure, mm Hg* | | |
Year	Active Treatment Group	Placebo Group	Difference (Active-Placebo)
	Systolic Blood Pressure		
Baseline	170.5 (9.5)	170.1 (9.2)	+0.4
1	142.5 (15.7)	156.5 (17.3)	−14.0
2	141.8 (17.1)	154.4 (18.7)	−12.6
3	142.4 (17.2)	155.0 (20.0)	−12.6
4	143.1 (18.0)	154.6 (19.8)	−11.5
5	144.0 (19.3)	155.1 (20.9)	−11.1
	Diastolic Blood Pressure		
Baseline	76.7 (9.6)	76.4 (9.8)	+0.3
1	69.5 (9.9)	73.4 (12.1)	−3.9
2	68.2 (10.9)	72.3 (12.0)	−4.1
3	68.0 (10.6)	72.1 (12.3)	−4.1
4	67.2 (11.6)	71.2 (12.6)	−4.0
5	67.7 (10.2)	71.1 (12.8)	−3.4

*Values are mean (SD).

taking antihypertensive medication was 1.24% and for those taking medication was 0.82%. Of those ineligible, 90% were excluded because of failure to meet blood pressure criteria.

Randomization and Baseline Characteristics of SHEP Participants

Randomization.—Stratified randomization by antihypertensive drug treatment status at initial contact and by center produced two SHEP groups—assigned to active treatment and placebo—comparable at baseline (Table 1).

Baseline Characteristics.—Mean age of participants was 72 years, 57% were women, and 14% were black (Table 1). Included among the whites were 204 Orientals (5% of whites), 84 Hispanics (2% of whites), and 41 classified as "other" (1% of whites). Of all participants, 1.4% reported a history of stroke, and 5% reported a history of myocardial infarction. On physical examination, 7% had carotid bruits. About 61% had an ECG abnormality. As a group, the cohort was overweight, with a body-mass index averaging 27.5 kg/m² (almost 30% overweight by actuarial

criteria).[43] Fewer than 1% had cognitive impairment, and about 11% manifested symptoms of depression based on standardized questionnaire criteria. Only 5% reported limitation in activities of daily living. Mean SBP was 170.3 mm Hg; mean DBP was 76.6 mm Hg. The distribution of SBP at baseline was 160 to 169 mm Hg, 57%; 170 to 179 mm Hg, 27%; 180 to 189 mm Hg, 10%; and greater than 190 mm Hg, 5%.

Antihypertensive Drug Treatment Status by Year of Follow-up

Active Treatment Group.—Most participants randomized to the active treatment group received active antihypertensive medication (either according to the SHEP protocol or by prescription) throughout the trial—89% of participants at year 3 and 90% of participants at year 5 (Table 2). About 3% of active treatment group participants were assigned to receive known active therapy because their blood pressure met the escape criteria; medication was stopped in 13% due to side effects. At the 5-year visit, of all participants in the active treatment group, 30% were receiving step 1, dose 1 medication only; 16% were receiving step 1, dose 2 medi-

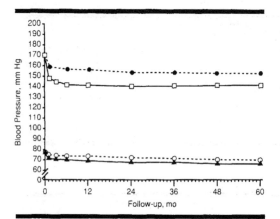

Fig 1. - Average systolic and diastolic blood pressure during the Systolic Hypertension in the Elderly Program follow-up plotted at 1, 3, 6, and 12 months and yearly therafter. Solid line with open squares indicates average systolic blood pressure for the active treatment group; broken line with closed circles, average systolic blood pressure for the placebo group; solid line with triangles, average diastolic blood pressure for the active treatment group; and broken line with open circles, diastolic blood pressure for the placebo group.

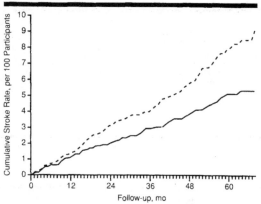

Fig 2.—Cumulative fatal plus nonfatal stroke rate per 100 participants in the active treatment (solid line) and placebo (broken line) groups during the Systolic Hypertension in the Elderly Program.

cation only; 11% were receiving step 2, dose 1 medication; 12% were receiving step 2, dose 2 medication; 21% were receiving other active medication; and 9% were receiving no antihypertensive drug. Thus, almost half of the participants were receiving the step 1 drug only, and more than two thirds of the participants were receiving the step 1 and/or step 2 drug only.

Placebo Group.—The majority of participants randomized to the placebo group continued to receive no active antihypertensive medication throughout the trial (Table 2). However, the percentage for whom active antihypertensive drug therapy was prescribed increased progressively, from 13% at year 1 to 33% at year 3 and 44% at year 5 (Table 2). Throughout the trial, about 15% of placebo group participants were assigned to receive active therapy because their blood pressure met the escape criteria (mostly due to DBP); medication was stopped in 7% due to side effects.

The proportion of participants receiving active antihypertensive medication was consistently higher throughout the trial for persons in the active treatment group than for those in the placebo group—89% vs 33% at 3 years and 90% vs 44% at 5 years (Table 2).

Mean SBP and DBP by Treatment Group and Year of Follow-up

Throughout the trial, the mean SBP of the active treatment group was substantially lower than at baseline, by about 26 mm Hg overall (Table 3 and Fig

Table 4.—Total (Nonfatal Plus Fatal) Stroke Rates by Treatment Group and Year of Follow-Up*

Year	Starting No.	No. of Events†	No. Unavailable for Follow-up	Cumulative Stroke Rate (SE), per 100 Participants
		Active Treatment Group		
1	2365	28	0	1.2 (0.2)
2	2316	22	0	2.1 (0.3)
3	2264	21	0	3.0 (0.4)
4	2153	18	0	4.0 (0.4)
5	1438	13	5	5.2 (0.5)
6‡	613	1	0	5.5 (0.6)
		Placebo Group		
1	2371	34	0	1.4 (0.2)
2	2308	42	0	3.2 (0.4)
3	2229	22	2	4.2 (0.4)
4	2131	34	2	6.0 (0.5)
5	1393	24	1	8.2 (0.7)
6	584	3	0	9.2 (0.9)

*For the active treatment group compared with the placebo group, χ^2(1 df) = 12.90, P = .0003; relative risk, 0.64 (95% confidence interval, 0.50 to 0.82).
†There were 103 total events (96 nonfatal and 10 fatal) in the active treatment group and 159 (149 nonfatal and 14 fatal) in the placebo group. Three participants in the active treatment group and four participants in the placebo group had both a nonfatal and a fatal stroke. Only the first event (nonfatal) was counted in the total number of events and in calculations of the cumulative stroke rate.
‡The last stroke occurred during the 67th month of follow-up.

Table 5.—Stroke Events by Treatment Group and Antihypertensive Medication Status at Initial Contact

Treatment Group	No. of Participants	No. of Events		Nonfatal Plus Fatal Stroke*
		Nonfatal Stroke	Fatal Stroke	
Not Receiving Antihypertensive Medication at Initial Contact				
Active	1584	64	5	67
Placebo	1577	88	11	96
Relative risk (95% confidence interval)†		0.69 (0.51-0.95)		
Receiving Antihypertensive Medication at Initial Contact				
Active	781	32	5	36
Placebo	794	61	3	63
Relative risk (95% confidence interval)‡		0.57 (0.38-0.85)		

*Three participants in the active treatment group and four participants in the placebo group had both a nonfatal and a fatal stroke. Only the first event (nonfatal) was counted in the total number of events.
†For the active treatment group compared with the placebo group, χ^2(1 df) = 5.40, P = .02.
‡For the active treatment group compared with the placebo group, χ^2(1 df) = 7.70, P = .01.

Table 6.—Morbidity and Mortality by Cause and Treatment Group

	Active Treatment Group (n=2365)	Placebo Group (n=2371)	Relative Risk (95% Confidence Interval)*
Nonfatal Events			
Stroke	96	149	0.63 (0.49-0.82)
Transient ischemic attack	62	82	0.75 (0.54-1.04)
Myocardial infarction†	50	74	0.67 (0.47-0.96)
Coronary artery bypass graft	30	47	0.63 (0.40-1.00)
Angioplasty	19	22	0.86 (0.47-1.59)
Left ventricular failure	48	102	0.46 (0.33-0.65)
Renal dysfunction	7	11	. . .
Fatal Events			
Total deaths	**213**	**242**	0.87 (0.73-1.05)
Total cardiovascular	90	112	0.80 (0.60-1.05)
Stroke	10	14	0.71 (0.31-1.59)
Total coronary heart disease	59	73	0.80 (0.57-1.13)
Sudden death (<1 h)	23	23	1.00 (0.56-1.78)
Rapid death (1-24 h)	21	24	0.87 (0.48-1.56)
Myocardial infarction	15	26	0.57 (0.30-1.08)
Other cardiovascular	21	25	0.87 (0.49-1.55)
Left ventricular failure	8	7	. . .
Other	13	18	0.71 (0.35-1.46)
Total noncardiovascular	109	103	1.05 (0.80-1.38)
Neoplastic disease	75	78	0.96 (0.70-1.31)
Renal disease	2	2	. . .
Diabetes mellitus	2	1	. . .
Gastrointestinal disease	2	2	. . .
Respiratory disease	6	5	. . .
Infectious disease	10	7	. . .
Accident, suicide, homicide	5	5	. . .
Other noncardiovascular	7	3	. . .
Indeterminate cause‡	14	27	. . .
Combined End Points			
Nonfatal myocardial infarction or coronary heart disease death	104	141	0.73 (0.57-0.94)
Fatal or nonfatal stroke, nonfatal myocardial infarction, or coronary heart disease death	199	289	0.67 (0.56-0.80)
Coronary heart disease§	140	184	0.75 (0.60-0.94)
Cardiovascular disease‖	289	414	0.68 (0.58-0.79)

*Relative risk assessments were done for all types of events except those with fewer than 20 events and indeterminate cause of death.

†Nonfatal myocardial infarction does not include silent myocardial infarction.

‡Results of death certificate coding for indeterminate causes according to the ninth revision of the *International Classification of Diseases, Adapted*, were as follows: stroke, two in the active treatment group and three in the placebo group; myocardial infarction, one in the placebo group; left ventricular failure, one in the placebo group; other cardiovascular disease, seven in the active treatment group and 10 in the placebo group; neoplasm, one in the active treatment group; respiratory disease, one in the placebo group; renal disease, one in the active treatment group; infectious disease, three in the placebo group; other noncardiovascular disease, one in the active treatment group and five in the placebo group; and unknown or no death certificate, one in the active treatment group and four in the placebo group.

§Coronary heart disease includes definite nonfatal or fatal myocardial infarction, sudden cardiac death, rapid cardiac death, coronary artery bypass graft, and angioplasty.

‖Cardiovascular disease includes definite nonfatal or fatal myocardial infarction, sudden cardiac death, rapid cardiac death, coronary artery bypass graft, angioplasty, nonfatal or fatal stroke, transient ischemic attack, aneurysm, and endarterectomy.

1). The mean DBP of the active treatment group was lower by about 9 mm Hg throughout the trial compared with baseline. For the placebo group, the mean SBP was consistently lower than at baseline, by about 15 mm Hg. The mean DBP of the placebo group was lower than at baseline by about 4 to 5 mm Hg. During the trial, the SHEP goal blood pressure was reached by 65% to 72% of persons in the active treatment group but only by 32% to 40% of those in the placebo group.

Mean SBP levels were substantially lower throughout the trial for the active treatment group than for the placebo group, by 11 to 14 mm Hg (Table 3 and Fig 1). Mean DBP was reduced more in the active treatment group than in the placebo group, by about 3 to 4 mm Hg.

Total Stroke Incidence

All Participants.—With a mean follow-up of 4.5 years, incident stroke, the primary end point of the trial, was diagnosed in 103 persons in the active treatment group and 159 persons in the placebo group (Table 4). By life table analyses, 5-year cumulative stroke rates were 5.2 per 100 participants for the active treatment group and 8.2 per 100 for the placebo group. The cumulative rates for the total period of follow-up (70 months) were 5.5 per 100 participants for the active treatment group and 9.2 per 100 for the placebo group. Based on proportional hazards regression analysis, relative risk was 0.64 (95% confidence interval [CI], 0.50 to 0.82; $P = .0003$) (Table 4 and Fig 2). The absolute reduction in 5-year risk of stroke was 30 events per 1000 participants. There were few stroke deaths—10 in the active treatment group and 14 in the placebo group. The cumulative difference in total stroke incidence rates, with rates lower in the active treatment group than in the placebo group, increased progressively over the 5 years of the trial (0.2, 1.1, 1.2, 2.0, and 3.0 events per 100 participants) (Table 4). Seventeen of 96 people in the active treatment group and 28 of 149 people in the placebo group who had a nonfatal stroke died during the trial—about 20% in each group.

By Age, Sex, Race, and Baseline SBP.—Stroke incidence was lower in those randomized to active treatment than in those randomized to placebo for all baseline age groups: 60 to 69 years, 34 vs 47 events; 70 to 79 years, 48 vs 74 events; and 80 years or older, 21 vs 38 events. A favorable effect of active treatment was also noted for three of the four major sex-race groups: white men, 39 vs 64 events; white women, 48 vs 66 events; and black women, seven vs 21 events. The apparent lack of any trend for the small number of black men was based on few events (nine vs eight events). With proportional hazards regression using SBP as a continuous variable, the favorable trend in stroke incidence for the active treatment compared with the placebo group prevailed irrespective of baseline SBP.

By Antihypertensive Drug Treatment Status at Initial Contact.—One of the two SHEP subgroup hypotheses was related to the effects of active treatment on participants receiving and not receiving antihypertensive medication at initial contact. Randomization was stratified by whether or not participants were receiving antihypertensive medication at initial contact. For the subgroup not receiving antihypertensive medication at initial contact, relative risk of stroke for active treatment compared with placebo was 0.69 (95% CI, 0.51 to 0.95) (Table 5). For participants receiving antihypertensive medication at initial contact, relative risk for stroke was 0.57 (95% CI, 0.38 to 0.85).

Thus, SHEP primary end point data indicate a high degree of consistency in favorable findings for the active treatment group.

Table 7.—Prevalence of Symptoms Ever Characterized as Troublesome or Intolerable by Treatment Group

Symptom	Prevalence, %		
	Active Treatment Group	Placebo Group	z
Cardiopulmonary			
Faintness on standing	12.8	10.6	2.3
Feelings of unsteadiness or imbalance	33.7	32.9	0.6
Loss of consciousness/passing out	2.2	1.3	2.6
Heart beating fast or skipping beats	7.2	8.3	-1.4
Heart beating unusually slowly	3.8	2.1	3.6
Chest pain or heaviness	28.0	21.3	5.3
Unusual shortness of breath	11.9	11.0	1.0
Unusual tiredness	25.8	23.8	1.6
Cold or numb hands	13.6	9.8	4.1
Ankle swelling	19.5	15.6	3.5
Psychosocial			
Unusual worry or anxiety	25.5	24.1	1.1
Trouble with memory/concentration	26.4	20.4	4.9
Depression that interfered with activities	10.7	10.6	0.1
Problems in sleeping	26.4	24.5	1.5
Nightmares	4.2	3.7	0.8
Problems in sexual function	4.8	3.2	2.9
Loss of appetite	6.4	5.5	1.4
Other			
Falls	12.8	10.4	2.5
Fractures	2.4	2.0	0.8
Muscle weakness or cramping	28.4	25.9	1.9
Unusual indigestion	10.3	8.9	1.6
Change in bowel habits	15.4	11.4	4.0
Excessive thirst	7.9	6.4	2.1
Nausea or vomiting	9.7	8.2	1.7
Tarry black stools or red blood in stools	2.2	2.1	0.3
Skin rash or bruising	12.5	10.6	2.0
Unusual joint pain	36.4	31.4	3.6
Severe headaches	7.8	8.7	-1.1
Waking frequently at night to urinate	14.4	12.4	2.0
Any specified problem	91.8	86.4	6.0
Any specified problem characterized as intolerable	28.1	20.8	5.9

Morbidity and Mortality From Cardiovascular and Noncardiovascular Causes

Nonfatal Cardiovascular Events.— The number of nonfatal cardiovascular events was consistently lower for active treatment than for placebo, with relative risks ranging from 0.46 for left ventricular failure to 0.86 for angioplasty (Table 6).

Hospitalizations and Nursing Home Admissions.— Hospitalizations for any reason were recorded for 1027 active treatment group participants (1976 admissions) and 1086 placebo group participants (2204 admissions). Skilled or intermediate care nursing home admissions were recorded for 52 active treatment group participants (58 admissions) and 58 placebo group participants (65 admissions).

Deaths by Cause.— The number of deaths was lower for active treatment than for placebo for mortality from all causes (213 vs 242 deaths), total cardiovascular causes (90 vs 112 deaths), and total coronary causes (59 vs 73 deaths) (range of relative risks, 0.80 to 0.87)

(Table 6). The difference observed in total deaths from coronary heart disease was largely due to the difference in the number of fatal myocardial infarctions. The number of deaths from neoplastic diseases, second only to cardiovascular disease as a main cause of mortality for SHEP participants, was similar (75 and 78 deaths) for the active treatment and placebo groups.

Combined Nonfatal and Fatal Cardiovascular Events.— Nonfatal and fatal major cardiovascular events were consistently lower for active treatment than placebo. All coronary heart disease events, nonfatal plus fatal, numbered 140 for the active treatment group and 184 for the placebo group (Table 6). By proportional hazards regression analysis, there were 25% fewer events in the active treatment group, with the 5-year absolute benefit estimated at 16 events per 1000 participants. All nonfatal and fatal cardiovascular events numbered 289 in the active treatment group and 414 in the placebo group. This represented 32% fewer events in the active treatment group, with the 5-year absolute benefit estimated at 55 events per

1000 participants.

Baseline ECG Abnormalities.— The end points for the second SHEP a priori subgroup hypothesis were the incidence of nonfatal myocardial infarction plus coronary death and the incidence of sudden and rapid death. The hypothesis dealt with the relationship of treatment assignment to risk of these events in persons with and without baseline ECG abnormalities. For the subgroup of people free of baseline ECG abnormalities, the relative risk of nonfatal myocardial infarction plus coronary death for active treatment compared with placebo was 0.83 (95% CI, 0.53 to 1.29). There were few events for the end point of sudden and rapid death—15 in the active treatment group and 10 in the placebo group. For participants with baseline ECG abnormalities, the relative risk of nonfatal myocardial infarction plus coronary death was 0.69 (95% CI, 0.50 to 0.94). For the end point of sudden and rapid death, there were 29 events in the active treatment group and 36 events in the placebo group.

The data regarding this subgroup hypothesis suggest benefit from active treatment for both those with and without baseline ECG abnormalities.

Adverse Effects

At baseline, the number of clinical complaints was comparable in the active treatment and placebo groups. During the trial, reported rates of certain problems were greater in the active treatment group than in the placebo group (Table 7).

During follow-up, serum potassium, uric acid, glucose, cholesterol, and sodium levels out of the specified ranges were reported more frequently in the active treatment group than in the placebo group (Table 8). During follow-up, the mean serum potassium concentration was lower in the active treatment group than in the placebo group; the mean serum uric acid, glucose, and cholesterol concentrations were higher in the active treatment group; and the mean serum sodium concentration was similar in the two groups (Table 8).

About 4% of persons in the active treatment and placebo groups met questionnaire referral criteria for expert evaluation of possible dementia (Table 9). For more than 90% of these people a referral was completed; the main reason for failure to achieve referral was participant refusal. Thirty-seven participants (1.6%) receiving active treatment and 44 (1.9%) receiving placebo had a diagnosis of dementia made and confirmed by the coding panel.

During the trial, 14% of persons in the active treatment group and 15% in the

Table 8.—Serum Biochemical Values by Treatment Group*

	Baseline		1 y			Ever		
	Active Treatment Group (n=2218)	Placebo Group (n=2202)	Active Treatment Group (n=1882)	Placebo Group (n=1821)	z	Active Treatment Group (n=2255)	Placebo Group (n=2189)	z
Serum potassium, mmol/L								
Mean ± SD	4.5 ± 0.5	4.5 ± 0.4	4.1 ± 0.5	4.4 ± 0.4	−25.2	...	...	...
% with values <3.2	0.1	0.0	1.0	0.1	3.8	3.9	0.8	6.7
Serum uric acid, µmol/L								
Mean ± SD	321.2 ± 83.3	315.2 ± 83.3	374.7 ± 101.1	327.1 ± 83.3	16.7	...	...	...
% with values ≥594.8	0.2	0.3	2.8	0.6	5.6	5.3	1.3	7.5
Serum glucose, mmol/L								
Mean ± SD	6.0 ± 1.9	6.0 ± 1.9	6.4 ± 2.4	6.1 ± 2.0	4.2	...	...	...
% with values ≥11.1	2.8%	3.0%	5.0	3.6	2.1	9.3	7.6	2.0
Serum cholesterol, mmol/L								
Mean ± SD	6.1 ± 1.2	6.1 ± 1.1	6.3 ± 1.2	6.1 ± 1.1	3.3	...	...	...
% with values ≥7.76	8.6	7.0	10.4	7.7	2.8	13.2	11.0	2.2
Serum sodium, mmol/L								
Mean ± SD	139.8 ± 2.5	139.6 ± 2.5	138.9 ± 3.0	139.6 ± 2.6	−7.6	...	...	...
% with values ≤130	0.3	0.2	1.8	0.4	4.4	4.1	1.3	5.6

*The number of participants in each treatment group and time period varied because of invalid values. We used the minimum number of participants.

Table 9.—Dementia and Depression by Treatment Group

	No. (%)	
	Active Treatment Group	Placebo Group
No. randomized	2365	2371
Dementia		
Qualified for referral	98 (4.1)	94 (4.0)
Referred	83 (3.5)	82 (3.5)
Positive diagnosis	37 (1.6)	44 (1.9)
Depression		
Qualified for referral	329 (13.9)	357 (15.1)
Referred	254 (10.7)	272 (11.5)
Positive diagnosis	104 (4.4)	112 (4.7)

placebo group met the questionnaire referral criteria for expert evaluation of possible depression (Table 9). For more than 75% of these people a referral was completed; the main reason for failure to achieve referral was participant refusal. Of participants in the two groups, 104 (4.4%) randomized to active treatment and 112 (4.7%) randomized to placebo had a diagnosis of depression.

COMMENT

The SHEP antihypertensive drug treatment regimen significantly reduced the risk of total stroke, the primary end point, in people aged 60 years and older with ISH. During the entire 70 months of study follow-up, the total stroke incidence was reduced by 36% in the active treatment group ($P = .0003$), and the absolute benefit estimated at 5 years was 30 events per 1000 participants. This result was observed even though about 35% of those assigned to placebo took known antihypertensive medications during the trial.

The incidence of nonfatal myocardial infarction (not including silent myocardial infarction) plus coronary death was 27% lower in the active treatment group than in the placebo group. This differ- ence was maintained when the combined coronary heart disease end point also included coronary angioplasty and coronary artery bypass grafting. For all cardiovascular events (289 in the active treatment and 414 in the placebo group), the reduction in incidence was 32% for the active treatment group. This is an absolute benefit at 5 years of 55 events per 1000 participants.

In addition to positive findings for the incidence of stroke, coronary heart disease, and cardiovascular disease, there was a favorable trend for total mortality. The death rate from all causes was 13% lower in the active treatment group than in the placebo group. (As anticipated by the SHEP design, given the sample size of the trial, this difference was not statistically significant.)

Favorable outcome for the active treatment group occurred for participants receiving and not receiving antihypertensive medication at initial contact. We recognize that persons not receiving antihypertensive drugs at initial contact might be more accurately characterized as individuals with ISH than those receiving such treatment.[1] However, we conclude that the SHEP drug regimen for reduction of blood pressure significantly reduced the incidence of stroke in persons aged 60 years and above with ISH, regardless of medication status at initial contact. Favorable findings are consistent for the active treatment group compared with the placebo group irrespective of age, sex-race, and baseline SBP.

The SHEP is the first trial to test the efficacy of antihypertensive drug treatment on clinical end points for persons with ISH. The significant positive outcome on its primary end point of stroke is consistent with the trend found in the SHEP pilot study.[44] The 36% reduction in stroke incidence is similar to that found in trials of drug therapy for diastolic hypertension, including the Hypertension Detection and Follow-up Program trial, the Medical Research Council trial, and 12 smaller trials combined.[45] Overall, these previous trials recorded a 42% reduction in stroke incidence (95% CI, 30% to 54%). Findings from SHEP and other trials suggest that antihypertensive drug treatment is broadly effective, with similar reductions in the stroke rate for people with either diastolic hypertension or ISH.

Moreover, the SHEP decrease of 27% in incidence of nonfatal myocardial infarction plus coronary heart disease death for the active treatment group is similar to results of the Hypertension Detection and Follow-up Program and greater than those in other trials. Combined results of all diastolic hypertension trials indicate that sustained net decrease in blood pressure recorded for active intervention produced an overall reduction in incidence of major coronary events of 14% (95% CI, 4% to 24%).[45]

For the coronary heart disease end point, SHEP recorded a favorable trend for participants with and without baseline ECG abnormalities. The SHEP medication regimen showed no evidence of adverse effect on coronary risk for people with baseline ECG abnormalities.[8,46,47] In fact, for SHEP participants with baseline ECG abnormalities (61% of those randomized), the incidence rate of nonfatal myocardial infarction plus coronary heart disease death was 31% lower for active treatment.

The positive SHEP outcome was achieved with minimum effective doses of antihypertensive drugs in a stepped-care regimen structured to achieve and maintain a goal blood pressure at least 20 mm Hg below baseline and below 160 mm Hg. It used low-dose chlorthalidone, 12.5 mg/d, as the step 1 medication. This was increased to a maximum of 25.0 mg/d if needed. The step 2 medication—usually low-dose atenolol, 25 mg/d, or, if atenolol was contraindicated, low-dose reserpine, 0.05 mg/d—was added as needed, and the dosage of either drug could have been doubled. High-level adherence to this regimen was maintained throughout the 5 years of the trial. Based on the effects of this regimen (plus regression to the mean and adaptation to clinic assessment), the average SBP of the active treatment group was lower during the trial by about 26 mm Hg, and it was about 11 mm Hg lower than the placebo group SBP. The average DBP of the active treatment group was about 3 to 4 mm Hg lower than the placebo group DBP. These data demonstrate an ability to achieve and sustain control of ISH in older persons with a low-dose, stepped-care drug regimen. This regimen was associated with only an infrequent excess of adverse effects and no evidence of increase in dementia or depression.

Also, the SHEP results may have implications for current uncertainties about optimal drug treatment regimens for diastolic hypertension, especially "mild" hypertension. The SHEP findings are congruent with the combined results of previous trials of drug treatment for diastolic hypertension in efficacy of preventing not only stroke but also coronary heart disease and all cardiovascular disease.[45] In all these trials an oral diuretic was the step 1 treatment drug. The SHEP was unique in two respects: it used low-dose chlorthalidone, and its participants were older people with ISH. The favorable SHEP results suggest that a low-dose oral diuretic, particularly chlorthalidone, may be as efficacious for step 1 drug treatment of high blood pressure as any other drug available. Data from large-scale, long-term randomized trials are not available—such data are needed.[48] The importance of this question is underscored by data on the comparative costs of oral diuretics and newer drugs.[49]

In conclusion, SHEP demonstrated significant efficacy of active antihypertensive drug treatment in preventing stroke in persons aged 60 years and older with ISH. This result was achieved (1) with use of stepped-care treatment, starting with low-dose chlorthalidone as the step 1 medication; (2) with the majority of participants assigned to active drug therapy being at or below the goal blood pressure; (3) with a low-order excess of adverse effects; and (4) with no excess incidence of depression or dementia. Favorable findings were demonstrated for multiple secondary end points of the trial, including the inci-

dence of major cardiac and cardiovascular events. These findings indicate a considerable potential for decreasing morbidity and disability by effective sustained drug treatment of ISH, given its prevalence and the high rates of cardiovascular diseases in those aged 60 years and older.

This study was supported by contracts with the National Heart, Lung, and Blood Institute and the National Institute on Aging. Drugs were supplied by the Lemmon Co, Sellersville, Pa; Wyeth Laboratories/Ayerst Laboratories, AH Robins Co, Richmond, Va; and Stuart Pharmaceuticals, Wilmington, Del.

References

1. The Systolic Hypertension in the Elderly Program (SHEP) Cooperative Research Group. Rationale and design of a randomized clinical trial on prevention of stroke in isolated systolic hypertension. *J Clin Epidemiol.* 1988;41:1197-1208.
2. Veterans Administration Cooperative Study Group on Antihypertensive Agents. Effects of treatment on morbidity in hypertension: results in patients with diastolic blood pressure averaging 115 through 129 mm Hg. *JAMA.* 1967;202:1028-1034.
3. Veterans Admistration Cooperative Study Group on Antihypertensive Agents. Effects of treatment on morbidity in hypertension, II: results in patients with diastolic blood pressure averaging 90 through 114 mm Hg. *JAMA.* 1970;213:1143-1152.
4. Wolff FW, Lindeman RD. Effects of treatment in hypertension: results of a controlled study. *J Chronic Dis.* 1966;19:227-240.
5. US Public Health Service Hospitals Cooperative Study Group. Treatment of mild hypertension: results of a 10 year intervention trial. *Circ Res.* 1977;40(suppl 1):98-105.
6. Veterans Administration/National Heart, Lung, and Blood Institute Study Group for Cooperative Studies on Antihypertensive Therapy: Mild Hypertension. Treatment of mild hypertension: preliminary results of a 2-year feasibility trial. *Circ Res.* 1977;40(suppl 1):180-187.
7. Veterans Administration/National Heart, Lung, and Blood Institute Study Group for Evaluating Treatment in Mild Hypertension. Evaluation of drug treatment in mild hypertension: VA-NHLBI feasibility trial. *Ann NY Acad Sci.* 1978;304:267-288.
8. Hypertension Detection and Follow-up Program Cooperative Group. Five-year findings of the Hypertension Detection and Follow-up Program, I: reduction in mortality in persons with high blood pressure, including mild hypertension. *JAMA.* 1979;242:2562-2571.
9. Hypertension Detection and Follow-up Program Cooperative Group. Five-year findings of the Hypertension Detection and Follow-up Program, II: mortality by race-sex and age. *JAMA.* 1979;242:2572-2576.
10. Hypertension Detection and Follow-up Program Cooperative Group. Five-year findings of the Hypertension Detection and Follow-up Program, III: reduction in stroke incidence among persons with high blood pressure. *JAMA.* 1982;247:633-638.
11. Hypertension Detection and Follow-up Program Cooperative Group. The effect of treatment on mortality in 'mild' hypertension. *N Engl J Med.* 1982;7:976-980.
12. Hypertension Detection and Follow-up Program Cooperative Group. Effect of stepped care on the incidence of myocardial infarction and angina pectoris. *Hypertension.* 1984;6(suppl 1):198-206.
13. Helgeland A. Treatment of mild hypertension: a 5-year controlled drug trial: the Oslo Study. *Am J Med.* 1980;69:725-732.
14. Leren P, Helgeland A. Oslo hypertension study. *Drugs.* 1986;31(suppl 1):41-45.
15. Australian National Blood Pressure Management Committee. The Australian therapeutic trial in mild hypertension. *Lancet.* 1980;1:1261-1267.
16. Medical Research Council Working Party. MRC trial of treatment of mild hypertension principal results. *BMJ.* 1985;291:97-104.
17. Hypertension-Stroke Cooperative Study Group. Effect of antihypertensive treatment on stroke recurrence. *JAMA.* 1974;229:409-418.
18. Barraclough M, Bainton O, Cochrane AL, et al. Control of moderately raised blood pressure: report of a cooperative randomized controlled trial. *BMJ.* 1973;3:434-436.
19. Amery A, Birkenhager W, Brixko P, et al. Mortality and morbidity results from the European Working Party on High Blood Pressure in the Elderly trial. *Lancet.* 1985;1:1349-1354.
20. Coope J, Warrender TS. Randomized trial of treatment of hypertension in the elderly in primary care. *BMJ.* 1986;293:1145-1151.
21. Carter AB. Hypotensive therapy in stroke survivors. *Lancet.* 1970;1:485-489.
22. Garland C, Barrett-Connor E, Suarez L, Criqui MH. Isolated systolic hypertension and mortality after age 60 years. *Am J Epidemiol.* 1983;118:365-376.
23. Probstfield JL, Furberg CD. Systolic hypertension in the elderly: controlled or uncontrolled. In: Frohlich ED, ed. *Preventive Aspects of Coronary Heart Disease.* Philadelphia, Pa: FA Davis Co Publishers; 1990:65-84.
24. Colandrea MA, Friedman GD, Nichaman MZ, Lynd CN. Systolic hypertension in the elderly: an epidemiologic assessment. *Circulation.* 1970;41:239-245.
25. Shekelle RB, Ostfeld AM, Klawans HL. Hypertension and risk of stroke in an elderly population. *Stroke.* 1974;5:71-75.
26. Dyer AR, Stamler J, Shekelle RB, Schoenberger JA, Farinaro E. Hypertension in the elderly. *Med Clin North Am.* 1977;61:513-529.
27. Rutan GH, Kuller LH, Neaton JD, Wentworth DN, McDonald RH, Smith WM. Mortality associated with diastolic hypertension and isolated systolic hypertension among men screened for the Multiple Risk Factor Intervention Trial. *Circulation.* 1988;77:504-514.
28. Stamler J, Neaton JD, Wentworth D. Blood pressure (systolic and diastolic) and risk of fatal coronary heart disease. *Hypertension.* 1989;13(suppl I):2-12.
29. Hulley SB, Furberg CD, Gurland B, et al. Systolic Hypertension in the Elderly Program (SHEP): antihypertensive efficacy of chlorthalidone. *Am J Cardiol.* 1985;56:913-920.
30. Borhani NO, Applegate WB, Cutler JA, et al. Systolic Hypertension in the Elderly Program (SHEP): baseline characteristics of the randomized sample, I: rationale and design. *Hypertension.* 1991;17(suppl II):2-15.
31. Black HR, Curb JD, Pressel S, Probstfield JL, Stamler J, eds. Systolic Hypertension in the Elderly Program (SHEP): baseline characteristics of the randomized sample. *Hypertension.* 1991;17(suppl II):1-171.
32. Wittes J, Davis B, Berge K, et al. Systolic Hypertension in the Elderly Program (SHEP): baseline characteristics of the randomized sample, X: analysis. *Hypertension.* 1991;17(suppl II):162-167.
33. Petrovitch H, Byington R, Bailey G, et al. Systolic Hypertension in the Elderly Program (SHEP): baseline characteristics of the randomized sample, II: screening and recruitment. *Hypertension.* 1991;17(suppl II):16-23.
34. Labarthe DR, Blaufox MD, Smith WM, et al. Systolic Hypertension in the Elderly Program (SHEP): baseline characteristics of the randomized sample, V: baseline blood pressure and pulse rate measurements. *Hypertension.* 1991;17(suppl II):62-76.
35. Weiler PG, Camel GH, Chiappini M, et al. Systolic Hypertension in the Elderly Program

Prevention of Stroke—SHEP Cooperative Research Group **3263**

(SHEP): baseline characteristics of the randomized sample, IX: behavioral characteristics. *Hypertension*. 1991;17(suppl II):152-161.

36. Gurland B, Golden RR, Teresi JA, Challop J: The SHORT-CARE: an efficient instrument for the assessment of depression, dementia and disability. *J Gerontol*. 1984;39:166-169.

37. *SHEP Manual of Operations*. Revised ed. Houston, Tex: University of Texas School of Public Health; 1990.

38. American Psychiatric Association, Committee on Nomenclature and Statistics. *Diagnostic and Statistical Manual of Mental Disorders, Revised Third Edition*. Washington, DC: American Psychiatric Association; 1987.

39. Mantel N. Evaluation of survival data and two new rank order statistics arising in its consideration. *Cancer Chemother Rep*. 1966;50:163-170.

40. Cox DR. Regression models and life tables. *J R Stat Soc B*. 1972;34:187-220.

41. Lan KKG, Wittes J. The B-value: a tool for monitoring data. *Biometrics*. 1988;44:579-585.

42. Davis BR, Hardy RJ. Upper bound for type I error and type II error rates in conditional power calculations. *Commun Stat*. 1990;19:3571-3584.

43. Hypertension Detection and Follow-up Program Cooperative Research Group. Mortality findings for stepped-care and referred-care participants in the Hypertension Detection and Follow-up Program, stratified by other risk factors. *Prev Med*. 1985;14:312-335.

44. Perry HM Jr, Smith WM, McDonald RH, et al. Morbidity and mortality in the Systolic Hypertension in the Elderly Program (SHEP) Pilot Study. *Stroke*. 1989;20:4-13.

45. Collins R, Peto R, MacMahon S, et al. Blood pressure, stroke and coronary heart disease, II: short-term reductions in blood pressure: overview of randomised drug trials in their epidemiological context. *Lancet*. 1990;335:827-838.

46. The Multiple Risk Factor Intervention Trial Research Group. Relationship among baseline resting ECG abnormalities, antihypertensive treatment and mortality in the Multiple Risk Factor Intervention Trial. *Am J Cardiol*. 1985;55:1-15.

47. Multiple Risk Factor Intervention Trial Research Group. Mortality after 10½ years for hypertensive participants in the Multiple Risk Factor Intervention Trial. *Circulation*. 1990;82:1616-1628.

48. Joint National Committee. The 1988 report of the Joint National Committee on Detection, Evaluation, and Treatment of High Blood Pressure. *Arch Intern Med*. 1988;148:1023-1038.

49. *Drug Topics Red Book*. Oradell, NJ: Medical Economics Books; 1990.

50. Kostis JB, Prineas R, Curb JD, et al. Systolic Hypertension in the Elderly Program (SHEP): baseline characteristics of the randomized sample, VIII: electrocardiographic characteristics. *Hypertension*. 1991;17(suppl II):123-151.

51. Prineas RJ, Crow RS, Blackburn H. *The Minnesota Code Manual of Electrocardiographic Findings: Standards and Procedures for Measurement and Classification*. Littleton, Mass: John Wright-PSG Inc; 1982.

SHEP COOPERATIVE GROUP INVESTIGATORS

Investigators at the 16 clinical centers and coordination and service centers of the SHEP Cooperative Group are listed below. For full membership in all SHEP subcommittees see Black et al.[31]

Albert Einstein College of Medicine, Bronx, NY.—M. Donald Blaufox, MD, PhD (*Principal Investigator*); William H. Frishman, MD; Gail Miller, RN; Maureen Magnani, RN; Sylvia Smoller, PhD; Zirel Sweezy.

Emory University School of Medicine, Atlanta, Ga.—W. Dallas Hall, MD (*Principal Investigator*); Sandy Biggio, RN, BSN; Margaret Chiappini, RN, BSN; Cori Hamilton; Margaret Huber, RN, BSN; Gail McCray; Deanne J Unger, RNC, BSN; Gary L. Wollam, MD.

Kaiser Permanente Center for Health Research, Portland, Ore.—Thomas M. Vogt, MD, MPH (*Principal Investigator*); Merwyn R. Greenlick, PhD; Stephanie Hertert; Patty Karlen, RN; Marlene McKenzie, RN, MN; Marcia Nielsen, RN, MN; Kathy Reavis, RN; Vicki Wegener, RN, FNP.

Medical Research Institute of San Francisco, Calif.—William McFate Smith, MD, MPH (*Principal Investigator*); Geri Bailey, RN; Philip Frost, MD; Jean Maier, RN; Ann Slaby; Jacqueline Smith, RN.

Miami (Fla) Heart Institute.—Fred Walburn, PhD (*Principal Investigator*); Maria Canosa-Terris, MD; Garcia Garrison, RN; Melissa Jones; Jeff Raines, PhD; Naidi Ritch; Avril Sampson, MD; Elisa Serantes, MD; Susan Surette.

Northwestern University Medical School, Chicago, Ill.—David Berkson, MD (*Principal Investigator*); Flora Gosch, MD; Joseph Harrington; Patricia Hershinow, RN; Josephine Jones; Angeline Merlo; Jeremiah Stamler, MD.

Pacific Health Research Institute, Honolulu, Hawaii.—Helen Petrovitch, MD (*Principal Investigator*); Sandra Akina, RN; J. David Curb, MD, MPH; Fred I. Gilbert, MD; Mary Hoffmeier, RN; Lei Honda-Sigall, RN.

Robert Wood Johnson Medical School, University of Medicine and Dentistry of New Jersey, Piscataway.—John B. Kostis, MD (*Principal Investigator*); Nora Cosgrove, RN; Susan Krieger, RN; Clifton R. Lacy, MD.

University of Alabama, Birmingham.—Richard M. Allman, MD (*Principal Investigator*); Ralph E. Allen, PA-C; Donna M. Bearden, MD; Lisa Carlisle; Vanessa P. Cottingham; Laura Farley, RN; Julia Hall; Glenn H. Hughes, PhD; Phillip Johnson; Linda Jones, CRNP; Laverne Parr; Pat Pierce; Harold W. Schnaper, MD.

University of California, Davis.—Nemat O. Borhani, MD, MPH (*Principal Investigator*); Patty Borhani; Alfredo Burlando, MD; Frances LaBaw, RN; Marshall Lee, MD; Sheila Lamé; Susan Pace, RN.

University of Kentucky Medical Center, Lexington.—Gordon P. Guthrie, Jr, MD (*Principal Investigator*); Jenny Brown; Jimmie Brumagen, RN; Ellen Christian, PA-C; Lynn Hanna, PA-C; Arlene Johnson, PhD; Jane Kotchen, MD; Theodore Kotchen, MD; William Markesbery, MD; Rita Schrodt, RN; John C. Wright, RN.

University of Minnesota, Minneapolis.—Richard H. Grimm, MD, PhD (*Principal Investigator*); Julie Levin; Mary Perron, RN; Alice Stafford.

University of Pittsburgh, Pa.—Lewis H. Kuller, MD, DrPH (*Co-Principal Investigator*); Robert McDonald, MD (*Co-Principal Investigator*); Shirley Arch (deceased); Gale Rutan, MD; Betsy Gahagan, RN; Jerry Noviello, PhD.

University of Tennessee, Memphis.—William B. Applegate, MD, MPH (*Principal Investigator*); Laretha Goodwin, RN, MBA; Stephen T. Miller, MD; Amelia Rose, RN; Alice Wallace, RN.

Washington University, St Louis, Mo.—H. Mitchell Perry, Jr, MD (*Principal Investigator*); Greta H. Camel, MD; Sharon Carmody; Jerome Cohen, MD; Judith Jensen, RN; Elizabeth Perry.

Yale University, New Haven, Conn.—Henry R. Black, MD (*Principal Investigator*); Diane Christianson, RN; Janice A. Davey, MSN; Charles K. Francis, MD; Linda Loesche.

School of Public Health, University of Texas Health Science Center at Houston (Coordinating Center).—C. Morton Hawkins, ScD (*Principal Investigator*); Barry R. Davis, MD; William S. Fields, MD; Darwin R. Labarthe, MD, PhD; Lemuel A. Moyé, MD, PhD; Sara Pressel, MS; Richard B. Shekelle, PhD.

Program Office, National Heart, Lung, and Blood Institute, Bethesda, Md.—*Project Officer:* Jeffrey L. Probstfield, MD; *Deputy Project Officer:* Eleanor Schron, RN, MS; *Former Project Officers:* Jeffrey A. Cutler, MD, MPH; Curt Furberg, MD, PhD; *Biostatistics Officers:* Edward Lakatos, PhD; Janet Wittes, PhD; *Contracting Officer:* C. Eugene Harris; *Contract Specialist:* Linda Gardner; *Other Key Personnel:* Thomas P. Blaszkowski, PhD; Clarissa Wittenberg, MSW.

National Institute on Aging, Bethesda, Md.—Evan Hadley, MD; J. David Curb, MD, MPH; Jack Guralnik, MD; Lot Page, MD (deceased); Teresa Radebaugh, ScD; Stanley Slater, MD; Richard Suzman, PhD.

Steering Committee.—Kenneth G. Berge, MD, Mayo Clinic, Rochester, Minn (*chair*).

Behavioral Assessment Subcommittee.—William B. Applegate, MD, MPH, (*chair*).

Clinic Coordinators Subcommittee.—Judith Jensen, RN (*chair*).

Drug Selection Working Group.—Robert McDonald, MD (*chair*).

Endpoints and Toxicity Subcommittee.—H. Mitchell Perry, Jr, MD (*chair*).

Operations and Medical Care Subcommittee.—Thomas M. Vogt, MD, MPH (*chair*).

Publications and Presentations Subcommittee.—Jeremiah Stamler, MD (*chair*).

Recruitment and Adherence Subcommittee.—Nemat O. Borhani, MD, MPH (*chair*).

Recruitment Coordinators Working Group.—Joseph Harrington (*chair*).

Scientific Review and Ancillary Studies Subcommittee.—W. Dallas Hall, MD (*chair*).

Executive Committee.—Kenneth G. Berge, MD (*chair*).

Data and Safety Monitoring Board.—James C. Hunt, MD (*Chair*), University of Tennessee. Memphis; C. E. Davis, PhD, University of North Carolina, Chapel Hill; Ray W. Gifford, Jr, MD. Cleveland (Ohio) Clinic Foundation; Millicent W. Higgins, MD, National Heart, Lung, and Blood Institute. Bethesda, Md; Adrian M. Ostfeld, MD, Yale University School of Medicine, New Haven, Conn; John W. Rowe, MD, Mt Sinai Medical Center, New York, NY; K. Warner Schaie, MD, Pennsylvania State University, State College; Herman A. Tyroler, MD, University of North Carolina, Chapel Hill; Jack P. Whisnant. MD, Mayo Clinic, Rochester, Minn; Joseph A. Wilber, MD, Atlanta, Ga.

Health Care Financing Administration, Washington, DC.—William Merashoff.

Drug Distribution Center, Perry Point, Md.—Richard Moss.

Central Chemical Laboratory (MetPath Laboratories, Teterboro, NJ).—S. Raymond Gambino, MD; Arlene Gilligan; Joseph E. O'Brien, MD; Nicholas Scalfratto; Elana Sommers.

Electrocardiographic Laboratory (University of Minnesota, Minneapolis).—Richard Crow, MD; Margaret Bodellan; Ronald J Prineas, MBBS, PhD.

Computed Tomogram Reading (University of Maryland, Baltimore).—L. Anne Hayman, MD; C. V. G. Krishna Rao, MD.

Consultants.—Marilyn Albert, PhD, Harvard Medical School and Massachusetts General Hospital, Boston; Lisa F. Berkman, PhD, Yale University, New Haven, Conn; Judith Challop-Luhr, PhD, Floral Park, NY; Debra Egan, MS, MPH, Washington, DC; June Gregonis, Duke University Medical Center, Durham, NC; Thomas R. Price, MD. University of Maryland Hospital, Baltimore; Ronald J. Prineas, MBBS, PhD, University of Miami, Fla; Kenneth A. Schneider, MD, Duke University Medical Center, Durham, NC; Philip Weiler, MD, University of California, Davis; Janet Wittes, PhD, Washington, DC.

Citation:

Are the results of this single preventive or therapeutic trial valid?

Was the assignment of patients to treatments randomised?
Was the randomisation list concealed?

Were all patients who entered the trial accounted for at its conclusion?
Were they analysed in the groups to which they were randomised?

Were patients and clinicians kept 'blind' to which treatment was being received?

Aside from the experimental treatment, were the groups treated equally?

Were the groups similar at the start of the trial?

Are the valid results of this randomised trial important?

SAMPLE CALCULATIONS (see pp134–40 of *Evidence-based Medicine*)

Occurrence of diabetic neuropathy		Relative risk reduction (RRR)	Absolute risk reduction (ARR)	Number needed to treat (NNT)
Usual insulin control event rate (CER)	Intensive insulin experimental event rate (EER)	$\dfrac{\text{CER} - \text{EER}}{\text{CER}}$	CER − EER	1/ARR
9.6%	2.8%	$\dfrac{9.6\% - 2.8\%}{9.6\%}$ $= 71\%$	9.6% − 2.8% $= 6.8\%$	1/6.8% $= 15$ pts

95% confidence interval (CI) on an NNT = 1 / (limits on the CI of its ARR) =

$$\pm 1.96\sqrt{\frac{\text{CER} \times (1-\text{CER})}{\text{\# of control pts}} + \frac{\text{EER} \times (1-\text{EER})}{\text{\# of exper. pts}}} = \pm 1.96\sqrt{\frac{0.096 \times 0.904}{730} + \frac{0.028 \times 0.972}{711}} = \pm 2.4\%$$

Are the valid results of this randomised trial important?

YOUR CALCULATIONS

		Relative risk reduction (RRR)	Absolute risk reduction (ARR)	Number needed to treat (NNT)
CER	EER	$\dfrac{\text{CER} - \text{EER}}{\text{CER}}$	CER – EER	1/ARR

Can you apply this valid, important evidence about therapy in caring for your patient?

Do these results apply to your patient?

Is your patient so different from those in the trial
that its results can't help you?

*How great would the potential benefit of therapy
actually be for your individual patient?*

Method I: **f**	Risk of the outcome in your patient, relative to patients in the trial. Expressed as a decimal: _____ NNT/f = ____/____ = _____ (NNT for patients like yours)
Method II: **1 / (PEER x RRR)**	Your patient's expected event rate if they received the control treatment: PEER: 1 / (PEER x RRR) = 1/_____ = _____ (NNT for patients like yours)

*Are your patient's values and preferences satisfied
by the regimen and its consequences?*

Do your patient and you have a clear assessment
of their values and preferences?

Are they met by this regimen and its consequences?

Additional notes

> **Citation:** SHEP Co-operative Research Group (1991) Prevention of stroke by antihypertensive drug treatment in older persons with isolated systolic hypertension. *JAMA.* **265:** 3255–64.

Are the results of this single preventive or therapeutic trial valid?

Was the assignment of patients to treatments randomised?	**Yes.**
Was the randomisation list concealed?	**Yes.**
Were all patients who entered the trial accounted for at its conclusion?	**Yes.**
Were they analysed in the groups to which they were randomised?	**Yes.**
Were patients and clinicians kept 'blind' to which treatment was being received?	**Yes, but may have been some unblinding because more of diuretic patients received potassium supplements.**
Aside from the experimental treatment, were the groups treated equally?	**Yes.**
Were the groups similar at the start of the trial?	**Yes, although some slight difference between groups in limitation of activities of daily living.**

Are the valid results of this randomised trial important?

SAMPLE CALCULATIONS (see pp134–40 of *Evidence-based Medicine*)

Occurrence of diabetic neuropathy		Relative risk reduction (RRR)	Absolute risk reduction (ARR)	Number needed to treat (NNT)
CER	EER	$\dfrac{CER - EER}{CER}$	CER − EER	1/ARR
9.6%	2.8%	$\dfrac{9.6\% - 2.8\%}{9.6\%}$ $= 71\%$	9.6% − 2.8% = 6.8%	1/6.8% = 15 pts

95% confidence interval (CI) on an NNT = 1 / (limits on the CI of its ARR) =

$$\pm 1.96 \sqrt{\frac{CER \times (1-CER)}{\# \text{ of control pts}} + \frac{EER \times (1-EER)}{\# \text{ of exper. pts}}} = \pm 1.96 \sqrt{\frac{0.096 \times 0.904}{730} + \frac{0.028 \times 0.972}{711}} = \pm 2.4\%$$

YOUR CALCULATIONS

		Relative risk reduction (RRR)	Absolute risk reduction (ARR)	Number needed to treat (NNT)
CER	EER	$\dfrac{CER - EER}{CER}$	CER – EER	1/ARR
0.07	0.04	$\dfrac{0.07 - 0.04}{0.07}$ = 57%	0.03	33

Can you apply this valid, important evidence about therapy in caring for your patient?

Do these results apply to your patient?

Is your patient so different from those in the trial that its results can't help you? | **No, he is similar to those included in the trial.**

How great would the potential benefit of therapy actually be for your individual patient?

Method I: **f**

Risk of the outcome in your patient, relative to patients in the trial.
Expressed as a decimal: **1.0**
NNT/f = **33/1 = 33**
(NNT for patients like yours)

Method II: **1 / (PEER x RRR)**

Your patient's expected event rate if they received the control treatment: PEER:
1 / (PEER x RRR) = 1/_____ = _____
(NNT for patients like yours)

Are your patient's values and preferences satisfied by the regimen and its consequences?

Do your patient and you have a clear assessment of their values and preferences? | **Needs to be assessed in each patient.**

Are they met by this regimen and its consequences? | **Needs to be assessed in each patient.**

Additional notes

HYPERTENSION – THERAPY WITH DIURETICS AND BETA BLOCKERS DECREASES THE RISK OF STROKE

Appraised by Sharon Straus: 1998.
Expiry date: 2000.

Clinical Bottom Line

Treatment of isolated systolic hypertension with diuretics and/or beta blockers decreases the risk of stroke in the elderly.

Citation

SHEP co-operative research group (1991) Prevention of stroke by antihypertensive drug treatment in older persons with isolated systolic hypertension. Final results of the systolic hypertension in the elderly program. (SHEP). *JAMA*. **265:** 3255–64.

Three-part Question

In a patient with hypertension, will therapy with diuretics decrease the risk of stroke and death?

Search Terms

'stroke' and 'hypertension' in *Best Evidence*.

The Study

1   Double-blinded concealed randomised controlled trial with intention-to-treat.
   Pts: 60 years with isolated systolic hypertension.

2   Control group (n = 2371; 2371 analysed): placebos.

3   Experimental group (n = 2365; 2365 analysed): four consecutive steps – chlorthalidone 12.5 mg/d; increase to chlorthalidone 25 mg/d; addition of atenolol 25 mg/d or reserpine 0.05 mg/d; increase to atenolol 50 mg/d or reserpine 0.1 mg/d. Goal of therapy was SBP <160 mmHg and a reduction in SBP of at least 20 mmHg. Any patient with sustained SBP >220 mmHg or DBP >90 mmHg was given active treatment.

The Evidence

Outcome	Time to outcome	CER	EER	RRR	ARR	NNT
Stroke	5 years	0.067	0.044	34%	0.023	43
95% confidence intervals				15% to 54%	0.107 to 0.036	28 to 100
Death	5 years	0.090	0.102	–13%	–0.012	–83
95% confidence intervals				–32% to 5%	–0.029 to 0.005	NNT = 209 to INF NNH = 35 to INF

Comments

1   Decreased risk of nonfatal MI or coronary heart disease death with treatment (RR 0.73 [0.57 to 0.94]).

2   Only enrolled 1% of the patients that were screened: included the very well elderly and therefore each clinician must assess each patient's individual baseline risk and individualise the NNT using this estimate.

3   At 5 years, 90% of the study group and 44% of controls were on active treatment and therefore the study likely underestimates the benefits of therapy since an intention-to-treat analysis was done.

4   Was there some unblinding because of the need for some patients (more often the ones receiving diuretics) to receive potassium supplements?

EBM SESSION

1

SECTION 2

Therapy
and asking
answerable
clinical
questions

PART A: Critical appraisal of a clinical article about therapy

You are responsible for a geriatric assessment program in your region that involves having people 75 years of age who live at home, seen by a multidisciplinary geriatric team. You are asked by a relative to see an 80-year old woman who lives by herself in the community and who has refused (on several occasions) to visit her GP. She has some difficulty with ambulating since she had a stroke five years previously. Her family is concerned because she has noted a decrease in visual acuity and hearing and they have noticed that her memory has declined. When you visit her, you find she is a very pleasant, independent woman who wants to know why you are there and how you can help her. You explain that you want to assess her physical and functional status and social situation because your aim is to help people maintain their independence in the community. She says, 'Prove it to me'.

You formulate the question: 'In an elderly patient who lives at home, does a comprehensive geriatric assessment decrease the risk of nursing home admission and improve functional status?'

Fortunately, you have brought your notebook computer with you which has the latest version of *Best Evidence* on it. You search *Best Evidence* using the term 'geriatric assessment' and find an abstract and commentary on an article by Stuck *et al.* which looks promising: *NEJM* (1995) **333:** 1184–9. You tell the patient that you will obtain this article from your office and will return to her with the evidence.

Read this article and decide:
1   Is the evidence from this randomised trial valid?
2   If valid, is this evidence important?
3   If valid and important, can you apply this evidence in caring for your patient?

If you want to read some strategies for answering these sorts of questions, you could have a look at pp 91–6, 133–41 and 166–72 in *Evidence-based Medicine.*

PART B: Asking answerable clinical questions

1   We illustrate the importance, strategies and tactics of formulating clinical questions and work with you on the three to four parts of the question.

2   Participants will break up into groups of two, discuss patients they cared for in the previous week, and generate questions they think are important concerning their patients' therapy, diagnosis and prognosis.

3   In larger groups, we review and refine the questions, and then keep track of them as possible questions to use in later sessions devoted to searching for the best evidence.

SPECIAL ARTICLES

A TRIAL OF ANNUAL IN-HOME COMPREHENSIVE GERIATRIC ASSESSMENTS FOR ELDERLY PEOPLE LIVING IN THE COMMUNITY

Andreas E. Stuck, M.D., Harriet U. Aronow, Ph.D., Andrea Steiner, Ph.D., Cathy A. Alessi, M.D., Christophe J. Büla, M.D., Marcia N. Gold, R.N., M.S.N., Karen E. Yuhas, R.N., M.P.H., Rosane Nisenbaum, Ph.D., Laurence Z. Rubenstein, M.D., and John C. Beck, M.D.

Abstract *Background and Methods.* The prevention of disability in elderly people poses a challenge for health care and social services. We conducted a three-year, randomized, controlled trial of the effect of annual in-home comprehensive geriatric assessments and follow-up for people living in the community who were 75 years of age or older. The 215 people in the intervention group were seen at home by gerontologic nurse practitioners who, in collaboration with geriatricians, evaluated problems and risk factors for disability, gave specific recommendations, and provided health education. The 199 people in the control group received their regular medical care. The main outcome measures were the prevention of disability, defined as the need for assistance in performing the basic activities of daily living (bathing, dressing, feeding, grooming, transferring from bed to chair, and moving around inside the house) or the instrumental activities of daily living (e.g., cooking, handling finances and medication, housekeeping, and shopping), and the prevention of nursing home admissions.

Results. At three years, 20 people in the intervention group (12 percent of 170 surviving participants) and 32 in the control group (22 percent of 147 surviving participants) required assistance in performing the basic activ-

ities of daily living (adjusted odds ratio, 0.4; 95 percent confidence interval, 0.2 to 0.8; P=0.02). The number of persons who were dependent on assistance in performing the instrumental activities of daily living but not the basic activities did not differ significantly between the two groups. Nine people in the intervention group (4 percent) and 20 in the control group (10 percent) were permanently admitted to nursing homes (P=0.02). Acute care hospital admissions and short-term nursing home admissions did not differ significantly between the two groups. In the second and third years of the study, there were significantly more visits to physicians among the participants in the intervention group than among those in the control group (mean number of visits per month, 1.41 in year 2 and 1.27 in year 3 in the intervention group, as compared with 1.11 and 0.92 visits, respectively, in the control group; P=0.007 and P=0.001, respectively). The cost of the intervention for each year of disability-free life gained was about $6,000.

Conclusions. A program of in-home comprehensive geriatric assessments can delay the development of disability and reduce permanent nursing home stays among elderly people living at home. (N Engl J Med 1995;333:1184-9.)

THE projected increase in the number of disabled older persons poses a challenge for health care and social services.[1] Comprehensive geriatric assessment has been used primarily for the evaluation and rehabilitation of chronically ill patients.[2,3] More effective preventive care for older persons might be achieved through a geriatric assessment in the home that was designed to detect and modify biologic, psychological, social, and environmental risk factors for disability.[4,5]

Comprehensive geriatric assessment directed toward rehabilitation has been shown to improve patients' outcomes, but this approach seems to be effective only in settings where the recommendations that arise from the assessment can be implemented.[3,6] Preventive home visits have been carried out in Denmark and the United

Kingdom, with variable results.[7-12] We conducted a randomized, controlled trial to test the effect of combining these two methods on the rate of disability in older persons living in the community.

METHODS

Study Participants

We used a voter-registration list to identify people in Santa Monica, California, who were 75 years of age or older and living at home.[13] Among the 966 persons contacted by telephone, 353 (37 percent) agreed to participate in the program. In addition, 86 persons were recruited by mail and 46 others asked to participate. Among these 485 subjects, 71 were excluded on the basis of the following a priori criteria: severe cognitive impairment (24 patients), language problems (18), plans to move to a nursing home (9), plans to move away (9), self-reported terminal disease (6), participation in another randomized trial (3), and severe functional impairment (2).

From December 1988 to June 1990, 215 of the participants were randomly assigned to the intervention group, and 199 to the usual-care (control) group. All participants gave written informed consent before being assigned to a group. Randomization was performed with sealed envelopes containing random numbers, with stratification according to age and sex. The study was approved by the institutional review committee at the University of California, Los Angeles.

Intervention

During the three-year study period, the people in the intervention group underwent annual comprehensive geriatric assessments per-

From the Multicampus Program in Geriatric Medicine and Gerontology, Department of Medicine (A.E.S., H.U.A., C.A.A., C.J.B., M.N.G., L.Z.R., J.C.B.), and the Department of Biostatistics, School of Public Health (R.N.), University of California, Los Angeles; the Department of Veterans Affairs Geriatric Research, Education, and Clinical Center, Sepulveda, Calif. (C.A.A., L.Z.R.); Senior Health and Peer Counseling, Santa Monica, Calif. (M.N.G., K.E.Y.); and the Institute for Health Policy Studies, University of Southampton, Southampton, United Kingdom (A.S.). Address reprint requests to Dr. Stuck at Morillonstr. 75, Zieglerspital, CH-3001 Bern, Switzerland.

Supported by grants from the W.K. Kellogg Foundation, the Swiss National Science Foundation (4032-35637), and Senior Health and Peer Counseling. Dr. Stuck was a Scholar of the Swiss Foundation for Biological and Medical Grants.

formed in their homes by gerontologic nurse practitioners. The assessment included a medical history taking, a physical examination, hematocrit and glucose measurements in blood samples obtained by finger stick, a dipstick urinalysis, and a mail-in fecal occult-blood test. The subjects were also evaluated for functional status,[14] oral health,[15] mental status (presence or absence of depression[16] and cognitive status[17]), gait and balance,[18] medications,[19] percentage of ideal body weight,[20] vision,[21] hearing,[21] extensiveness of social network,[13] quality of social support,[13] and safety in the home and ease of access to the external environment. The nurse practitioners discussed each case with the study geriatricians, developed rank-ordered recommendations, and conducted in-home follow-up visits every three months to monitor the implementation of the recommendations, make additional recommendations if new problems were detected, and facilitate compliance. If additional contact was considered necessary, the nurse practitioner telephoned the participant or was available by telephone. All the participants were encouraged to take an active role in their care and to improve their ability to discuss problems with their physicians. Only in complex situations did the nurse practitioners or study physicians contact the patients' physicians directly.[22]

Of the 215 people in the intervention group, 13 were never seen by nurse practitioners: 3 died and 10 declined to be visited. The remaining 202 people received a mean ($\pm$SD) of 10.9$\pm$3.2 visits during the three-year study period. Forty-nine people did not complete the program because they died (20 participants), moved out of the area (13), moved to a nursing home (9), or refused to continue (7).

Each year, participants were given an average of 5.9 recommendations about self-care (e.g., physical exercise, sleep, management of urinary incontinence, nutrition, use of over-the-counter medications, compliance with regimens involving prescription medications, use of aids and devices, and safety in the home; accounting for 51 percent of all recommendations), 3.3 recommendations to discuss new problems or potentially suboptimal therapy with their personal physicians (29 percent), and 2.3 recommendations involving the use of community services (20 percent). On average, the participants adhered to 47 percent of all recommendations, did not adhere to 39 percent, and partly adhered to 14 percent (usually those involving changes in long-term behavior, such as nutrition or exercise). In addition, the nurse practitioners reinforced primary and secondary prevention by monitoring the frequency of regular dental care, vaccinations, eye examinations, breast self-examination, Pap smears, and mammographic screening.[23] Telephone interviews of a subgroup of 102 participants in the intervention group revealed that 99 percent of them were satisfied with the program and that 84 percent would have liked to continue the preventive home visits after the completion of the study.

Outcome Measures

Before randomization and annually thereafter for three years, patients were seen at home by trained interviewers not involved in the intervention who used a structured interview format. Information was collected on the basic activities of daily living (bathing, dressing, feeding, grooming, transferring from bed to chair, and moving around inside the house),[14] instrumental activities of daily living (e.g., cooking, handling finances and medication, housekeeping, and shopping),[14] and combined basic and instrumental activities,[24] and a hierarchical score was calculated.[25] Analysis of disability-free survival was based on date-of-death information and on functional status (basic activities of daily living) at base line and at three years. Information on hospital admissions was based on a systematic review of the participants' names and Social Security and Medicare numbers at all local hospitals.

In telephone interviews conducted every four months by the independent interviewers, the participants or, in cases of a severe decline in health, predesignated proxies provided information about nursing home admissions and use of community services. The nursing home information was systematically verified by reviewing hospital-discharge data and contacting local nursing homes.

Information on visits to physicians was obtained from Medicare claims files and local health maintenance organizations. Nursing home stays were classified as either permanent or short-term. Stays were deemed permanent if the participants remained for 100 days or more or if they were admitted for terminal care. Short-term stays were defined as lasting fewer than 100 days and ending with a discharge to the participant's home.[26]

Statistical Analysis

All analyses were based on a priori hypotheses, with functional status and nursing home admissions as the primary outcomes.[27,28] Base-line characteristics of the participants were added to the intention-to-treat models of the effects of the intervention. Proportional-hazards models were used for survival data. For functional status at three years, we used repeated-measures regression analyses, adding functional status at one and two years to the models after ascertaining that there was no interaction between time and treatment effect. In addition, standard and polychotomous logistic-regression techniques were used. The effects of the intervention on the number of hospital admissions for acute care, short-term nursing home admissions, and visits to physicians were based on multivariate Poisson regression models corrected for overdispersion.[29]

We estimated the required sample size needed for an alpha level of 0.05 (two-tailed) on the basis of data from similar trials.[2,7,8] According to this estimate, a sample of 200 persons in each group was sufficient (with a statistical power of 0.8) to detect a 40 percent reduction in the number of persons with disability and a 25 percent change in the number of acute hospital admissions, with a marginal ability (statistical power of 0.5) to detect a 50 percent reduction in nursing home admissions.

Sensitivity analyses were conducted by repeating the analyses with the base-line characteristics of the participants excluded, as well as outliers, if appropriate. In addition, analyses of functional status were repeated, with imputed (estimated) values used for missing data. The imputed estimates were derived from the known base-line and outcome data, with the use of maximum-likelihood techniques and simulations.[30]

To determine whether certain subgroups benefited more from the intervention than others, age, sex, functional status, self-perceived health, and education were added as covariate by treatment interaction terms to the covariate models. All statistical tests were two-sided, with a P value of 0.05 considered to indicate statistical significance.

RESULTS

The base-line characteristics of the people in the intervention and control groups were similar (Table 1). Survival at three years was also similar in the two groups, with 24 deaths (11 percent) in the intervention group and 26 (13 percent) in the control group (odds ratio, 0.8; 95 percent confidence interval, 0.5 to 1.5; P=0.8). Vital status and location of residence were known for all participants at three years.

Functional Status

At three years, the people in the intervention group had a higher mean functional status than those in the control group (Table 2). The detailed results of a hierarchical analysis are shown in Table 3. With independence as the reference state, the odds of being dependent on assistance in the basic activities of daily living at three years were significantly lower in the intervention group than in the control group (adjusted odds ratio, 0.4; 95 percent confidence interval, 0.2 to 0.8; P=0.02; P=0.03 for the unadjusted odds ratio). The odds of being dependent on assistance only for the instrumental

---

activities of daily living were similar in the two groups (odds ratio, 1.1; 95 percent confidence interval, 0.6 to 2.0; P = 0.8).

Analyses in which values were imputed for missing functional-status measures yielded somewhat larger estimates of the treatment effect for all measures than did the primary analysis. The primary analysis may therefore understate the true effect of treatment on functional status.

Permanent Nursing Home Admissions

During the three-year period, 9 persons in the intervention group and 20 in the control group were permanently admitted to nursing homes (odds ratio for the intervention group as compared with the control group, 0.4; 95 percent confidence interval, 0.2 to 0.9; P = 0.02) (Table 4). There were approximately one

Table 2. Mean Functional-Status Score among the Surviving Participants at Three Years, According to Intention-to-Treat Analysis.*

FUNCTIONAL-STATUS SCORE	INTERVENTION GROUP (N = 170)	CONTROL GROUP (N = 147)	DIFFERENCE IN SCORES (INTERVENTION GROUP VS. CONTROL GROUP)	P VALUE
	mean (95% CI)			
Basic ADL†	96.8 (94.8–98.8)	95.4 (93.4–97.4)	+1.4 (−0.3 to +3.1)	0.1
Instrumental ADL‡	72.3 (69.0–75.6)	69.3 (66.0–72.6)	+3.0 (+0.6 to +5.4)	0.02
Basic and instrumental ADL	75.6 (73.2–77.9)	72.7 (70.2–75.2)	+2.9 (+0.4 to +5.4)	0.03

*Data are based on reports by 287 study participants and 30 proxies (in most cases, a spouse or close relative) during the home interview at three years. Data were not available for 45 persons in the intervention group (24 died, 14 refused, and 7 moved away) and 52 in the control group (26 died, 21 refused, and 5 moved away). Results have been adjusted for age, sex, whether the subject lived alone, base-line self-perceived health, and base-line functional status. ADL denotes activities of daily living, and CI confidence interval. All scores are on a scale of 0 to 100, with 100 representing the highest functional status.

†As defined in Table 1.

‡Instrumental ADL include cooking, handling finances, handling medication, engaging in "handyman" work, housekeeping, doing laundry, shopping, using the telephone, and using public or private transportation.

sixth as many nursing home days in the intervention group as in the control group. Six people in the intervention group and seven in the control group were living in nursing homes at the three-year follow-up. Information on functional status at three years was available for four surviving people in each group; all eight were dependent on assistance in performing the basic activities of daily living.

Acute Care Hospital Admissions

The intervention did not have a significant effect on the number of admissions to acute care hospitals or the number of short-term nursing home stays (Table 4). Eighteen percent of the study participants in the intervention group and 21 percent of those in the control group were admitted at least once to an acute care hospital in the first year; 21 and 20 percent, respectively, were admitted at least once in the second year; and 24 and 25 percent, respectively, were admitted at least once in the third year. The mean length of stay per acute care admission was 6.3 days in the intervention group and 5.1 days in the control group (P = 0.7, by the polychotomous logistic-regression analysis). With self-reported hospital admissions outside the study area added to the data in Table 4, the estimated number of hospital days per 100 subjects per year was 203 for the intervention group and 180 for the control group.

Although there was no overall effect of the intervention on hospital admissions, we performed an exploratory analysis to determine whether the intervention was associated with an increased or decreased number of admissions among certain subgroups of study participants. A polychotomous logistic-regression analysis showed that the intervention was associated with a decreased number of short stays (i.e., those lasting one to seven days) among persons with fair or poor self-perceived health (odds ratio, 0.4; 95 percent confidence interval, 0.2 to 1.0; P = 0.05) and among those with less than a high-school education (odds ratio, 0.3; 95 percent confidence interval, 0.1 to 1.0; P = 0.04). None of

Table 1. Base-Line Characteristics of the Study Participants, According to the Original Group Assignment.*

CHARACTERISTIC BEFORE RANDOM ASSIGNMENT	INTERVENTION GROUP (N = 215)	CONTROL GROUP (N = 199)
Age — yr	81.0±3.9	81.4±4.2
Women — no. (%)	149 (69)	141 (71)
Living alone — no. (%)	140 (65)	125 (63)
Completed high school — no. (%)	173 (80)	151 (76)
Annual income <$11,000 — no. (%)†	82 (38)	74 (37)
Mean score for self-perceived health‡	3.2±1.2	3.1±1.2
Independence in basic ADL — no. (%)	196 (91)	183 (92)
Depression score§	2.8±2.7	3.1±2.9
Regular exercise — no. (%)	142 (66)	116 (58)
Current nonsmoker — no. (%)	198 (92)	184 (92)
No. of medications	4.9±2.8	4.6±3.1
No. of visits to physicians in previous month	1.3±1.4	1.1±1.6
CHARACTERISTIC AT INITIAL GERIATRIC ASSESSMENT¶		
Arterial hypertension — no. (%)	67 (33)	—
Poor vision — no. (%)	34 (17)	—
Poor hearing — no. (%)	61 (30)	—
Impaired gait and balance — no. (%)	20 (10)	—
Underweight — no. (%)	14 (7)	—
Overweight — no. (%)	54 (27)	—
In-home hazard — no. (%)	61 (30)	—

*Plus–minus values are means ±SD. Basic ADL denotes basic activities of daily living (bathing, dressing, feeding, grooming, transferring from bed to chair, and moving around inside the house).

†An annual income of $11,000 is considered the poverty line.

‡The rating scale for self-perceived health ranges from 5 (excellent) to 1 (poor).

§The Geriatric Depression Scale, short form, ranges from 0 to 15, with a score above 5 indicating probable depression.

¶Data are missing for 13 persons who dropped out of the study before the assessment could be performed. Assessments were not performed in the control group. Arterial hypertension was defined as >160 mm Hg systolic or >90 mm Hg diastolic. Poor vision was defined as <20/50 in the better eye. Poor hearing was defined as 1000 or 2000 Hz not heard at 40 dB in the better ear. Impairment in gait and balance was defined as a score <23 on a scale of 0 to 28, with 28 representing the best result.[18] Underweight was defined as 20 percent below average body weight, and overweight as 20 percent above average body weight.[20]

Table 3. Functional Status (Dependence or Independence) of the Surviving Participants at Three Years, According to Intention-to-Treat Analysis.

FUNCTIONAL STATUS	INTERVENTION GROUP (N = 170)	CONTROL GROUP (N = 147)	ODDS RATIO (95% CI)*	P VALUE
	no. of persons (%)			
Dependent on assistance in basic ADL†	20 (12)	32 (22)	0.4 (0.2–0.8)	0.02
Dependent on assistance in instrumental but not basic ADL‡	39 (23)	28 (19)	1.1 (0.6–2.0)	0.8
Independent §	111 (65)	87 (59)	—	—

*Odds ratios are based on a polychotomous logistic-regression analysis adjusted for age, sex, whether the subject lived alone, base-line self-perceived health, and base-line functional status, with independent persons as the reference group. The odds ratios are for the intervention group, as compared with the control group. CI denotes confidence interval.

†Dependence was defined as requiring assistance in at least one of the basic activities of daily living (ADL; defined in Table 1).

‡Dependence was defined as independence in basic ADL but a need for assistance in at least one of the instrumental ADL (defined in Table 2).

§Independence was defined as a need for no assistance in either basic or instrumental ADL.

the subgroups of the intervention group had significant increases in admissions to acute care hospitals.

Use of Community Services

The intervention was not associated with changes in the use of in-home and supportive services. Study participants in the intervention group were more likely than those in the control group to use services promoting socialization, such as college courses for older persons or a friendly-visitor program (Table 5).

Visits to Physicians

In the second and third years, the people in the intervention group had significantly more outpatient visits than those in the control group (Table 6). Exploratory subgroup analyses showed that this effect was more pronounced among the study participants with symptoms of depression (P = 0.03). The intervention was also associated with a reduction in the proportion of persons who did not visit a physician in a 12-month period. Nine percent of the study participants in the intervention group, as compared with 16 percent of those in the control group, did not visit a physician during the third year of follow-up (P = 0.04).

Cost Estimates

The approximate yearly cost of the intervention can be derived from the costs of the program itself, including the costs for personnel (1.0 full-time-equivalent nurse practitioner and 0.1 full-time-equivalent geriatrician per 136 persons), supplies, travel, and overhead (estimated at $48,000 per 100 persons); the mar-

ginal costs for the increased number of visits to physicians (estimated at $18,000 per 100 persons); and the marginal savings from the decreased number of permanent-stay nursing home days (estimated at $42,000 per 100 persons), resulting in a net cost of $24,000 per 100 persons. Acute care hospital admissions and short-term nursing home stays are not included in this calculation, because they did not differ significantly between the two groups.

The effect of the intervention on health-related outcomes can be summarized in two ways: by estimating the number of disability-free years gained by the intervention (4.1 years per 100 persons per year during the 3-year follow-up), or by calculating the number of permanent-stay nursing home days avoided (692 days [820 − 128] per year) (Table 4). On the basis of these estimates, the cost for each disability-free year of life gained was approximately $6,000. The cost of preventing one day of a permanent stay in a nursing home was $35.

DISCUSSION

We found that a three-year program of comprehensive in-home geriatric assessments resulted in a significant reduction in the number of persons who required assistance in performing the basic activities of daily living and a significant reduction in the number of permanent nursing home admissions. Although it is not possible to determine whether the reduction in disability was responsible for the reduction in nursing home admissions, such a relation is likely. The intervention emphasized reducing the risk factors for disability. There was no measurable increase in the use of supportive home care services. All participants living in nursing homes at three years were dependent on assistance in performing the basic activities of daily living. These findings suggest that the prevention of declines in functional status at least partially explains the reduction in nursing home admissions.

Table 4. Hospital and Nursing Home Admissions during the Three-Year Follow-up Period, According to Intention-to-Treat Analysis.*

TYPE OF ADMISSION	INTERVENTION GROUP (N = 215)	CONTROL GROUP (N = 199)	ADJUSTED ODDS RATIO OR RELATIVE RISK (95% CI)†	P VALUE
Permanent nursing home				
No. of persons admitted (%)	9 (4)	20 (10)	OR = 0.4 (0.2–0.9)	0.02
No. of days/100 persons/yr	128	820		
Acute care hospital				
No. of persons admitted at least once (%)	99 (46)	93 (47)	RR = 1.0 (0.8–1.4)	0.8
No. of days/100 persons/yr	197	160		
Short-term nursing home				
No. of persons admitted at least once (%)	27 (13)	31 (16)	RR = 0.9 (0.6–1.4)	0.6
No. of days/100 persons/yr	89	111		

*Nursing home data are based on information reported by the study participants, with verification from secondary sources. Permanent and short-term admissions are defined in the text. Hospital data are based on systematic reviews of admissions to local hospitals.

†Results have been adjusted for age, sex, base-line self-perceived health, and base-line functional status. The odds ratio (OR) is based on a multivariate logistic-regression analysis, and the relative risks (RR) are based on multivariate Poisson analyses corrected for overdispersion. The odds ratio and relative risks are for the intervention group, as compared with the control group. CI denotes confidence interval.

It is unlikely that these results have been affected by missing information. Sensitivity analyses indicated that the 12 percent rate of missing data on functional status at three years did not result in an overestimation of treatment effects and may actually have caused an underestimation of these effects (data not shown).

The intervention was not a substitute for usual care (medical and social services) but instead was integrated with such care. It was therefore not unexpected that, as a result of the recommendations by the nurse practitioners, the people in the intervention group consulted their physicians more frequently than the people in the control group. To calculate the overall cost of the intervention, we included the cost of these additional visits to physicians.

Two European trials have found that preventive home visits can reduce the number of admissions to acute care hospitals.[8,11] Our intervention did not appear to have this effect. We hypothesize that this may reflect a balance between two opposite effects of the intervention. It is likely that among study participants with previously unrecognized or suboptimally managed problems, hospital admissions increased, whereas among other participants, unnecessary admissions were prevented.

As compared with the U.S. population of persons 75 years old or older living at home, our study group had a higher educational level, a lower mortality rate, and a lower rate of acute care hospital admissions, with a higher proportion of persons living alone.[31,32] Caution should therefore be used in generalizing our results to different groups, such as older persons in rural communities or those with a lower level of education.

The results of our study support the view that a program of comprehensive in-home geriatric assessments may help prevent disability, but it cannot be determined from our results which components of the program are most important. Other controlled studies have shown that preventive home visits without an an-

nual comprehensive geriatric assessment,[7-12] a one-time in-home geriatric assessment with follow-up,[33] regular telephone follow-up,[34] or health promotion[35-37] may improve outcomes in the elderly. It is unlikely that the social contacts provided by our intervention resulted in the observed effects, since social contacts alone have been shown to be ineffective.[38] The reasons for the benefits of this approach are being explored so that even more effective strategies can be developed.[39]

We are indebted to Thomas Belin, Ph.D., David Draper, Ph.D., Robert Elashoff, Ph.D., Gerhard Gillmann, and Christoph E. Minder, Ph.D., for statistical analyses; to Kristiana Raube, Ph.D., for her many valuable contributions during the first two years of the project; to Kathryne Barnowski, R.N., Bernice Bratter, Guillemette Epailly, Roslyn Fanello, R.N., Michele Kemp, Harriet Kossove, Pat McDonough, R.N., M.S., Heather Murray, John Oishi, Alisha Oropallo, Hans Pensel, Maridette Schloe, Rose Udin, and Scott Watanabe; and to the participants for their help in carrying out this study.

Table 6. Mean Number of Visits to Physicians per Month, According to Intention-to-Treat Analysis.*

Year	Intervention Group		Control Group		Adjusted Relative Risk (95% CI)†	P Value
	No. of Persons	Mean No. of Visits	No. of Persons	Mean No. of Visits		
1	207	1.27	185	1.03	1.1 (1.0–1.3)	0.1
2	199	1.41	180	1.11	1.2 (1.1–1.4)	0.007
3	191	1.27	162	0.92	1.4 (1.1–1.6)	0.001

*Data are based on Medicare claims data and on records of health maintenance organizations. Persons who had died, moved permanently to nursing homes, or moved out of the area were excluded from the analysis. In addition, 22 persons (8 in the intervention group and 14 in the control group) were excluded because reliable data on the number of visits to physicians were not available.

†Relative risks (based on a multivariate Poisson analysis corrected for overdispersion) have been adjusted for age, sex, membership in a health maintenance organization, base-line self-perceived health, and base-line functional status. Relative risks are for the intervention group, as compared with the control group. CI denotes confidence interval.

Table 5. Use of Community Services during the Three-Year Follow-up Period, According to Intention-to-Treat Analysis.*

Type of Service	Intervention Group (N = 215)	Control Group (N = 199)	P Value
	no. of persons (%)		
In-home and supportive services			
Care management†	43 (20)	33 (17)	0.4
Home health care	27 (13)	17 (9)	0.2
Homemaker	24 (11)	28 (14)	0.4
Meals on wheels	23 (11)	18 (9)	0.6
Personal care	20 (9)	24 (12)	0.4
Services promoting socialization			
College courses for senior citizens	45 (21)	23 (12)	0.01
Friendly visitors‡	23 (11)	7 (4)	0.01
Community transportation	57 (27)	36 (18)	0.04

*Data are based on reports provided by the study participants at one or more of the interviews conducted every four months during the three-year follow-up period.

†Formerly known as case management.

‡Denotes a home-based program that schedules social visits by volunteers with elderly persons.

REFERENCES

1. Jackson ME, Siu AL, Drugovich ML, et al. Alternative projections of the disabled elderly population: report to the Administration on Aging. Washington, D.C.: Public Health Service, 1991.
2. Rubenstein LZ, Josephson KR, Wieland GD, English PA, Sayre JA, Kane RL. Effectiveness of a geriatric evaluation unit: a randomized clinical trial. N Engl J Med 1984;311:1664-70.
3. Stuck AE, Siu AL, Wieland GD, Adams J, Rubenstein LZ. Comprehensive geriatric assessment: a meta-analysis of controlled trials. Lancet 1993;342:1032-6.
4. Verbrugge LM, Jette AM. The disablement process. Soc Sci Med 1994;38:1-14.
5. Guralnik JM, Ferrucci L, Simonsick EM, Salive ME, Wallace RB. Lower-extremity function in persons over the age of 70 years as a predictor of subsequent disability. N Engl J Med 1995;332:556-61.
6. Reuben DB, Borok GM, Wolde-Tsadik G, et al. A randomized clinical trial of comprehensive geriatric assessment in the care of hospitalized patients. N Engl J Med 1995;332:1345-50.
7. Vetter NJ, Jones DA, Victor CR. Effect of health visitors working with elderly patients in general practice: a randomised controlled trial. BMJ 1984;288:369-72.
8. Hendriksen C, Lund E, Strømgård E. Consequences of assessment and intervention among elderly people: a three year randomised controlled trial. BMJ 1984;289:1522-4.
9. Carpenter GI, Demopoulos GR. Screening the elderly in the community: controlled trial of dependency surveillance using a questionnaire administered by volunteers. BMJ 1990;300:1253-6.
10. McEwan RT, Davison N, Forster DP, Pearson P, Stirling E. Screening elderly people in primary care: a randomised controlled trial. Br J Gen Pract 1990;40:94-7.
11. Pathy MSJ, Bayer A, Harding K, Dibble A. Randomised trial of case finding and surveillance of elderly people at home. Lancet 1992;340:890-3.

12. Vetter NJ, Lewis PA, Ford D. Can health visitors prevent fractures in elderly people? BMJ 1992;304:888-90.
13. Rubenstein LZ, Aronow HU, Schloe M, et al. A home-based geriatric assessment, follow-up and health promotion program: design, methods, and baseline findings from a 3-year randomized clinical trial. Aging Clin Exp Res 1994;6:105-20.
14. Lawton MP, Moss M, Fulcomer M, Kleban MH. A research and service oriented multilevel assessment instrument. J Gerontol 1982;37:91-9.
15. Atchinson KA, Dolan TA. Development of the Geriatric Oral Health Assessment Index. J Dent Educ 1990;54:680-7.
16. Sheikh JI, Yesavage JA. Geriatric Depression Scale (GDS): recent evidence and development of a shorter version. In: Brink TL, ed. Clinical gerontology: a guide to assessment and intervention. New York: Haworth Press, 1986:165-73.
17. Kahn RL, Goldfarb AI, Pollack M. Peck A. Brief objective measures for the determination of mental status in the aged. Am J Psychiatry 1960;117:326-8.
18. Tinetti ME, Baker DI, McAvay G, et al. A multifactorial intervention to reduce the risk of falling among elderly people living in the community. N Engl J Med 1994;331:821-7.
19. Stuck AE, Beers MH, Steiner A, Aronow HU, Rubenstein LZ, Beck JC. Inappropriate medication use in community-residing older persons. Arch Intern Med 1994;154:2195-200.
20. Master AM, Lasser RP, Beckman G. Tables of average weight and height of Americans aged 65 to 94 years. JAMA 1960;172:658-63.
21. Lachs MS, Feinstein AR, Cooney LM Jr, et al. A simple procedure for general screening for functional disability in elderly patients. Ann Intern Med 1990;112:699-706.
22. Büla CJ, Alessi CA, Aronow HU, et al. Cooperation of community physicians with a program of in-home comprehensive geriatric assessment. J Am Geriatr Soc 1995;43:1016-20.
23. Preventive Services Task Force. Guide to clinical preventive services: an assessment of the effectiveness of 169 interventions. Baltimore: Williams & Wilkins, 1989.
24. Kempen GI, Suurmeijer TP. The development of a hierarchical polychotomous ADL-IADL scale for noninstitutionalized elders. Gerontologist 1990; 30:497-502.
25. Spector WD. Katz S, Murphy JB, Fulton JP. The hierarchical relationship between activities of daily living and instrumental activities of daily living. J Chronic Dis 1987;40:481-9.
26. Liu K, McBride T, Coughlin T. Risk of entering nursing homes for long versus short stays. Med Care 1994;32:315-27.
27. Afifi AA, Clark V. Computer-aided multivariate analysis. 2nd ed. New York: Van Nostrand Reinhold, 1990.
28. Dawson-Saunders B, Trapp RG. Basic and clinical biostatistics. Norwalk, Conn.: Appleton & Lange, 1990.
29. Overdispersion. In: Aitkin M, Anderson D, Francis B, Hinde J. Statistical modelling in GLIM. Vol. 4 of Oxford Statistical Science Series. Oxford, England: Oxford University Press, 1989:223.
30. Rubin DB. Multiple imputation for nonresponse in surveys. New York: John Wiley, 1987.
31. National Center for Health Statistics, Adams PF, Benson V. Current estimates from the National Health Interview Survey, 1989. Vital and health statistics. Series 10. No. 176. Washington, D.C.: Government Printing Office, 1990. (DHHS publication no. (PHS) 90-1504.)
32. National Center for Health Statistics, Benson V, Marano MA. Current estimates from the National Health Interview Survey, 1992. Vital and health statistics. Series 10. No. 189. Washington, D.C.: Government Printing Office, 1994. (DHHS publication no. (PHS) 94-1517.)
33. Fabacher D, Josephson K, Pietruszka F, Linderborn K, Morley JE, Rubenstein LZ. An in-home preventive assessment program for independent older adults: a randomized controlled trial. J Am Geriatr Soc 1994;42: 630-8.
34. Wagner EH, LaCroix AZ, Grothaus L, et al. Preventing disability and falls in older adults: a population-based randomized trial. Am J Public Health 1994;84:1800-6.
35. Hall N, De Beck P, Johnson D, Mackinnon K. Randomized trial of a health promotion program for frail elders. Can J Aging 1992;11:72-91.
36. van Rossum E, Frederiks CMA, Philipsen H. Portengen K, Wiskerke J, Knipschild P. Effects of preventive home visits to elderly people. BMJ 1993;307:27-32.
37. Wasson J, Gaudette C, Whaley F, Sauvigne A, Baribeau P, Welch HG. Telephone care as a substitute for routine clinic follow-up. JAMA 1992;267: 1788-93.
38. Clarke M, Clarke SJ, Jagger C. Social intervention and the elderly: a randomized controlled trial. Am J Epidemiol 1992;136:1517-23.
39. Stuck AE. Gafner Zwahlen H, Neuenschwander BE, Meyer Schweizer RA, Bauen G, Beck JC. Methodologic challenges of randomized controlled studies on in-home comprehensive geriatric assessment: the EIGER project. Aging Clin Exp Res 1995;7:218-23.

The *Journal*'s E-Mail Addresses:

For letters to the Editor:
letters@edit.nejm.org

For information about submitting material for Images in Clinical Medicine:
images@edit.nejm.org

For information about the status of a submitted manuscript:
status@edit.nejm.org

Citation:

Are the results of this single preventive or therapeutic trial valid?

Was the assignment of patients to treatments randomised?
Was the randomisation list concealed?

Were all patients who entered the trial accounted for at its conclusion?
Were they analysed in the groups to which they were randomised?

Were patients and clinicians kept 'blind' to which treatment was being received?

Aside from the experimental treatment, were the groups treated equally?

Were the groups similar at the start of the trial?

Are the valid results of this randomised trial important?

SAMPLE CALCULATIONS (*see* pp134–40 of *Evidence-based Medicine*)

Occurrence of diabetic neuropathy		Relative risk reduction (RRR)	Absolute risk reduction (ARR)	Number needed to treat (NNT)
Usual insulin control event rate (CER)	Intensive insulin experimental event rate (EER)	$\dfrac{CER - EER}{CER}$	CER − EER	1/ARR
9.6%	2.8%	$\dfrac{9.6\% - 2.8\%}{9.6\%}$ $= 71\%$	9.6% − 2.8% $= 6.8\%$	1/6.8% $= 15$ pts

95% confidence interval (CI) on an NNT = 1 / (limits on the CI of its ARR) =

$$+/-1.96 \sqrt{\frac{CER \times (1-CER)}{\text{\# of control pts}} + \frac{EER \times (1-EER)}{\text{\# of exper. pts}}} = +/-1.96 \sqrt{\frac{0.096 \times 0.904}{730} + \frac{0.028 \times 0.972}{711}} = +/-2.4\%$$

Are the valid results of this randomised trial important?

YOUR CALCULATIONS

		Relative risk reduction (RRR)	Absolute risk reduction (ARR)	Number needed to treat (NNT)
CER	EER	$\dfrac{CER - EER}{CER}$	CER – EER	1/ARR

Can you apply this valid, important evidence about therapy in caring for your patient?

Do these results apply to your patient?

Is your patient so different from those in the trial that its results can't help you?

How great would the potential benefit of therapy actually be for your individual patient?

Method I: **f**	Risk of the outcome in your patient, relative to patients in the trial. Expressed as a decimal: _____ NNT/f = ____/____ = _____ (NNT for patients like yours)
Method II: **1 / (PEER x RRR)**	Your patient's expected event rate if they received the control treatment: PEER: 1 / (PEER x RRR) = 1/_____ = _____ (NNT for patients like yours)

Are your patient's values and preferences satisfied by the regimen and its consequences?

Do your patient and you have a clear assessment of their values and preferences?

Are they met by this regimen and its consequences?

Additional notes

Citation: Stuck AE, Aronow HU, Steiner A *et al.* (1995) A trial of annual in-home comprehensive geriatric assessments for elderly people living in the community. *NEJM*. 333: 1184–9.

Are the results of this single preventive or therapeutic trial valid?

Was the assignment of patients to treatments randomised?	**Yes.**
Was the randomisation list concealed?	**Yes.**

Were all patients who entered the trial accounted for at its conclusion?	**Yes.**
Were they analysed in the groups to which they were randomised?	**Yes.**

Were patients and clinicians kept 'blind' to which treatment was being received?	**Interviewers who did the follow-up assessments were blinded.**

Aside from the experimental treatment, were the groups treated equally?	**Yes.**

Were the groups similar at the start of the trial?	**Yes.**

Are the valid results of this randomised trial important?

SAMPLE CALCULATIONS (*see* pp134–40 of *Evidence-based Medicine*)

Occurrence of diabetic neuropathy		Relative risk reduction (RRR)	Absolute risk reduction (ARR)	Number needed to treat (NNT)
CER	EER	$\dfrac{\text{CER} - \text{EER}}{\text{CER}}$	CER – EER	1/ARR
9.6%	2.8%	$\dfrac{9.6\% - 2.8\%}{9.6\%}$ = 71%	9.6% – 2.8% = 6.8%	1/6.8% = 15 pts

95% confidence interval (CI) on an NNT = 1 / (limits on the CI of its ARR) =

$$+/-1.96\sqrt{\frac{\text{CER} \times (1-\text{CER})}{\text{\# of control pts}} + \frac{\text{EER} \times (1-\text{EER})}{\text{\# of exper. pts}}} = +/-1.96\sqrt{\frac{0.096 \times 0.904}{730} + \frac{0.028 \times 0.972}{711}} = +/-2.4\%$$

YOUR CALCULATIONS (admission to long-term nursing homes)

		Relative risk reduction (RRR)	Absolute risk reduction (ARR)	Number needed to treat (NNT)
CER	EER	$\dfrac{\text{CER} - \text{EER}}{\text{CER}}$	CER – EER	1/ARR
0.10	0.04	58%	0.06	17

Can you apply this valid, important evidence about therapy in caring for your patient?

Do these results apply to your patient?

Is your patient so different from those in the trial that its results can't help you?	**No, this patient is similar.**

How great would the potential benefit of therapy actually be for your individual patient?

Method I: **f**	Risk of the outcome in your patient, relative to patients in the trial. Expressed as a decimal: **1.0** NNT/f = **17/1 = 17** (NNT for patients like yours)
Method II: **1 / (PEER x RRR)**	Your patient's expected event rate if they received the control treatment: PEER: 1 / (PEER x RRR) = 1/_____ = _____ (NNT for patients like yours)

Are your patient's values and preferences satisfied by the regimen and its consequences?

Do your patient and you have a clear assessment of their values and preferences?	**Needs to be assessed in each patient.**
Are they met by this regimen and its consequences?	**Needs to be assessed in each patient.**

Additional notes

GERIATRIC ASSESSMENT – IMPROVES FUNCTIONAL STATUS AND DECREASES NURSING HOME ADMISSIONS

Appraised by Sharon Straus: 1998.
Expiry date: 2000.

Clinical Bottom Line

Geriatric assessment decreases admissions to long-term nursing homes and improves functional status.

Citation

Stuck AE, Aronow HU, Steiner A *et al.* (1995) A trial of annual in-home comprehensive geriatric assessments for elderly people living in the community. *NEJM.* **333**: 1184–9.

Three-part Question

In an elderly patient who lives at home, does a comprehensive geriatric assessment decrease the risk of nursing home admission and improve functional status?

Search Terms

'geriatric assessment' in *Best Evidence.*

The Study

1 Single-blinded randomised controlled trial without intention-to-treat. Pts: >75 years of age who lived at home.

2 Control group (n = 199; 199 analysed): usual care by their physicians.

3 Experimental group (n = 215; 215 analysed): annual assessments in their homes from gerontologic nurse practitioners. Assessments included medical history, physical exam, lab tests, determinations of functional and mental status, oral health, gait and balance, medications, vision, hearing, social network and support, home safety and external access.

The Evidence

Outcome	Time to outcome	CER	EER	RRR	ARR	NNT
Long-term nursing home admission	3 years	0.101	0.042	58%	0.059	17
95% confidence intervals				9% to 100%	0.009 to 0.109	9 to 108
Admission to acute care hospital	3 years	0.467	0.460	1%	0.007	143
95% confidence intervals				−19% to 22%	−0.089 to 0.103	NNT = 10 to Inf NNH = 11 to Inf

Comments

1 Cost of intervention included in this paper but may differ according to your location.

2 These patients had higher education level, lower mortality rate and lower rate of acute care hospital admission – you therefore need to compare this to your own population to assess applicability.

3 Uncertain which components of the geriatric assessment are the most important and have the greatest impact on maintaining independence.

Your turn: case-presentations

- Take one of your patients who presented an important problem in therapy, diagnosis, prognosis, or harm.

- Formulate that problem into a three-part question (the patient, the manoeuvre and the outcome), based on what you learn from Session 1.

- Do a search for the best evidence based on what you learn from Sessions 3–5 (lots of help available from us or the library team).

- Critically appraise that evidence for its validity, importance, and usefulness.

- Integrate that appraisal with clinical expertise and summarise it (in a one-pager if you wish).

- Present it to the rest of us at one of the final sessions. (Certificates will be given to presenters.)

PART A — Critical appraisal of a clinical article about the diagnosis of anaemia

You admit a well 75-year old woman with community acquired pneumonia. She responds nicely to appropriate antibiotics but her haemoglobin remains at 100 g/l with a mean cell volume of 80. Her peripheral blood smear shows hypochromia, she is otherwise well, and is on no incriminating medications. You contact her GP and find out that her haemoglobin was 105 g/l six months ago. She has never been investigated for anaemia. You discuss this patient with your registrar and debate the use of ferritin in the diagnosis of iron deficiency anaemia. You admit to yourself that you are unsure how to interpret a ferritin result and how precise and accurate a serum ferritin is for diagnosing iron deficiency anaemia.

You therefore form the question: 'In an elderly woman with hypochromic, microcytic anaemia, can a low ferritin diagnose iron deficiency anaemia?' You order a ferritin and head for the library (10 days later it comes back at 40 µg/l).

Searching *Best Evidence* on disk with the single word 'ferritin' yielded a very encouraging meta-analysis of 55 studies and a nice individual study, but your library didn't carry either journal. You perform a MEDLINE search using the MeSH terms 'ferritin' and 'sensitivity and specificity' and find an article on diagnosing iron deficiency anaemia in the elderly published in a journal that your library does take: *Am J Med* (1990) **88:** 205–9.

Read this article and decide:
1 Are the results of this diagnostic article valid?
2 Are the valid results of this diagnostic study important?
3 Can you apply this valid, important evidence about a diagnostic test in caring for your patient?

If you want to read some strategies for answering these sorts of questions, you could have a look at pp 81–4, 118–28 and 159–63 in *Evidence-based Medicine*.

PART B — Searching the evidence-based journals

We show you how to search the electronic version of two journals: *ACP Journal Club* (ACPJC) and *Evidence-based Medicine*. The contents of these journals are available on disk as *Best Evidence*. This requires a computer with a CD slot and can be ordered from the BMJ Publishing Group, PO Box 295, London WC1H 9TE; Tel: 0171 387 4499 (subscriptions); Fax: 0171 383 6662; email: bmjsubs@dial.pipex.com.

You might try out searching these evidence-based journals for answers to some of the questions you generated last week.

Diagnosis of Iron-Deficiency Anemia in the Elderly

GORDON H. GUYATT, M.D., CHRISTOPHER PATTERSON, M.D., MAHMOUD ALI, M.D., JOEL SINGER, Ph.D., MARK LEVINE, M.D., IRENE TURPIE, M.D., RALPH MEYER, M.D., *Hamilton, Ontario, Canada*

PURPOSE: To determine the value of serum ferritin, mean cell volume, transferrin saturation, and free erythrocyte protoporphyrin in the diagnosis of iron-deficiency anemia in the elderly.

PATIENTS AND METHODS: We prospectively studied consecutive eligible and consenting anemic patients over the age of 65 years, who underwent blood tests and bone marrow aspiration. The study consisted of 259 inpatients and outpatients at two community hospitals in whom a complete blood count processed by the hospital laboratory demonstrated previously undiagnosed anemia (men: hemoglobin level less than 12 g/dL; women: hemoglobin level less than 11.0 g/dL).

RESULTS: Thirty-six percent of our patients had no demonstrable marrow iron and were classified as being iron-deficient. The serum ferritin was the best test for distinguishing those with iron deficiency from those who were not iron-deficient. No other test added clinically important information. The likelihood ratios associated with the serum ferritin level were as follows: greater than 100 μg/L, 0.13; greater than 45 μg/L but less than or equal to 100 μg/L, 0.46; greater than 18 μg/L but less than or equal to 45 μg/L, 3.12; and less than or equal to 18 μg/L, 41.47. These results indicate that values up to 45 μg/L increase the likelihood of iron deficiency, whereas values over 45 μg/L decrease the likelihood of iron deficiency. Seventy-two percent of those who were not iron-deficient had serum ferritin values greater than 100 μg/L, and in populations with a prevalence of iron deficiency of less than 40%, values of greater than 100 μg/L reduce the probability of iron deficiency to under 10%. Fifty-five percent of the iron-deficient patients had serum ferritin values of less than 18 μg/L, and in populations with a prevalence of iron deficiency of greater than 20%, values of less than 18 μg/L increase the probability of iron deficiency to over 95%.

CONCLUSION: In a general geriatric medical population such as ours, with a prevalence of iron deficiency of 36%, appropriate use of serum ferritin determination would establish or refute a diagnosis of iron deficiency without a bone marrow aspiration in 70% of the patients.

Anemia is an extremely common problem in the elderly, and next to anemia of chronic disease, iron deficiency is the most common cause. Iron-deficiency anemia is important to diagnose because appropriate iron therapy may improve symptoms, inappropriate iron therapy may cause clinically important side effects, and iron deficiency may be a marker for occult gastrointestinal pathology.

Although bone marrow aspiration provides a definitive diagnosis of iron-deficiency anemia, the value of less invasive tests of iron stores in general populations has been well established [1–9]. Serum ferritin and transferrin saturation are the tests most commonly used. Because bone marrow aspiration can be painful and is more expensive than laboratory tests, the procedure is often reserved for patients in whom the diagnosis remains in doubt after noninvasive test results are available.

Our interest in the investigation of iron deficiency in the elderly was stimulated by a clinical impression that application of cutoff points for laboratory tests for the diagnosis of iron deficiency derived from younger populations was misleading in a geriatric population. There are a number of reasons why results found in younger populations may not apply to the elderly. The iron-binding capacity decreases with aging [10,11], and is affected by factors such as malnutrition and chronic disease, which have a higher prevalence in the elderly [12]. Serum ferritin levels increase with aging [13], and may be elevated by acute and chronic inflammatory conditions [14,15]. One small study has suggested that measurements of transferrin saturation and serum ferritin in elderly anemic patients with and without iron deficiency differ significantly from those found in younger patients [16]. These problems have led to varying recommendations regarding the interpretation of results of noninvasive tests of iron stores in the elderly [16–18].

There are other reasons why further study of the diagnosis of anemia is warranted. First, investigations to date have generally used a single cut-point, and reported on the sensitivity and specificity of the tests. This approach discards valuable information. Use of multiple cut-points, with determination of likelihood ratios associated with each range of results, provides additional information for the clinician [19]. Second, statistically reliable determination of the best single test, and whether additional useful information could

From the Department of Medicine (GHG, CP, MA, ML, IT, RM), the Department of Clinical Epidemiology and Biostatistics (GHG, ML), and the Department of Family Practice (JS), McMaster University, Hamilton, Ontario, Canada. This work was supported in part by the Ontario Ministry of Health. Dr. Guyatt is a Career Scientist of the Ontario Ministry of Health. Requests for reprints should be addressed to Gordon H. Guyatt, M.D., Department of Clinical Epidemiology and Biostatistics, McMaster University Health Sciences Centre, Room 2C12, 1200 Main Street West, Hamilton, Ontario, Canada, L8N 3Z5. Manuscript submitted July 13, 1989, and accepted in revised form November 14, 1989.
Current addresses: Department of Medicine, Chedoke Hospital, Hamilton, Ontario, Canada (CP); Department of Pathology, St. Joseph's Hospital, Hamilton, Ontario, Canada (MA); Department of Medicine, St. Joseph's Hospital, Hamilton, Ontario, Canada (IT); Department of Family Medicine, McMaster University Health Sciences Centre, Hamilton, Ontario, Canada (JS); and Department of Medicine, Henderson General Hospital, Hamilton, Ontario, Canada (ML, RM).

TABLE I

Reasons For Exclusion of Patients Found To Be Anemic on at Least One Hemoglobin Determination

Reason for Exclusion	Number of Patients Excluded
Patient judged too ill, demented, or terminal	212
Patient or family refused consent for bone marrow aspiration	200
Not anemic on second hemoglobin determination	200
Recent transfusion	152
Previous bone marrow aspiration had revealed diagnosis	108
Institutionalized	95
Miscellaneous	108
Total	1,075

TABLE II

Final Primary Diagnosis of Anemia

Diagnosis	Number of Patients
Iron-deficiency anemia	94
Anemia of chronic disease	113
Megaloblastic anemia	21
Multiple myeloma	4
Sideroblastic anemia	3
Dysmyeloplastic	3
Other*	21
Total	259

* Includes patients with leukemia, hemolytic anemia, hypoplastic and aplastic marrow, renal failure, and hypothyroidism, and those with inadequate information for definitive diagnosis.

be gained from performing a second or third test, has seldom been investigated. Third, other tests (including the free erythrocyte protoporphyrin) have been suggested as being potentially useful in confirming the diagnosis of iron-deficiency anemia, but have not been adequately studied.

Because of the frequency of anemia in the elderly, and because of the difficulties in performing bone marrow aspirations in all anemic patients, we believed it important to determine the accuracy of less invasive laboratory tests commonly used to assess iron stores. Our criterion or gold standard for the diagnosis of iron deficiency was the results of the bone marrow aspiration.

PATIENTS AND METHODS

Consecutive patients over the age of 65 years presenting to Chedoke Hospital in Hamilton, Ontario, between January 1984 and March 1988 with anemia (in men, hemoglobin 12.0 g/dL or less on two consecutive occasions; in women, 11.0 g/dL or less) were identified through the hospital laboratory. An additional much smaller group of patients admitted to St. Joseph's Hospital in Hamilton under one of the co-investigators and meeting study criteria were also included. We excluded institutionalized patients, those with recent blood transfusions or documented acute blood loss, or those whose participation in the study was judged unethical by their attending physician (for reasons such as impending death or severe dementia). Detailed criteria for definition of "too ill," "impending

death," or "severe dementia" were not established. Rather, we relied on physician judgment in these areas. Similarly, we relied on physicians for the appropriate level of encouragement to patient participation when obtaining informed consent.

All patients had the following laboratory tests: hemoglobin, mean red cell volume (MCV), red cell distribution width (RDW), serum iron, iron-binding capacity, serum ferritin, and red cell protoporphyrin. The complete blood count was carried out using a Coulter S $+IV^{TM}$ (Coulter Electronics, Miami, Florida). Serum iron and iron-binding capacity were measured according to the methods of the International Committee for Standardization in Haematology [20]. Serum ferritin was determined using a radioimmunoassay described in detail previously [21]. Red cell protoporphyrin was measured using a previously described micromethod [22]. A bone marrow aspiration was undertaken and the findings were interpreted by a hematologist (M.A.) who was unaware of the results of the laboratory tests. The bone marrow slides were air-dried, fixed with methanol, and stained with Prussian blue [23]. Results of the first 65 marrow aspirations were also interpreted by a second hematologist (also unaware of the laboratory test findings), and discrepancies resolved by consensus. The results of the aspiration were classified as iron absent, reduced, present, or increased. After interpreting the marrow aspiration results, the hematologist reviewed all relevant clinical information and made a final decision regarding the cause(s) of the anemia. Anemia of chronic disease was diagnosed when the iron present in the reticuloendothelial cells (fragments) was increased and the number of sideroblasts (red cells containing iron granules) was decreased. The increase in reticuloendothelial iron was defined as iron granules covering 50% of all the fragments observed, and a decrease in sideroblasts was confirmed when iron granules were present in less than 20% of the red cells.

Statistical Methods

Receiver operating characteristic (ROC) curves for each test were generated. The area under the curves was compared using the method of Hanley and McNeil [24]. Since the ROC curves in this study were all generated from the same cohort of patients, we used the correction factor, which reflects the correlation between the tests [25]. Using the same cut-points, likelihood ratios for each category were calculated.

To determine the independent contribution of each test to the diagnosis, and whether a combination of tests could improve diagnostic accuracy, stepwise logistic regression procedures were used. The status of iron stores (present or absent) was used as the dependent variable, and the values of the diagnostic tests (dichotomized using the cut-point that maximized accuracy) as the independent variables.

Chance-corrected agreement between the two hematologists who interpreted the marrow aspiration results was calculated using a weighted kappa, with quadratic weights.

RESULTS

Aside from providing more precise estimates of the likelihood ratios, inclusion of 25 patients from St. Joseph's Hospital had no systematic effect on the results of any analysis. Thus, these patients will not be identi-

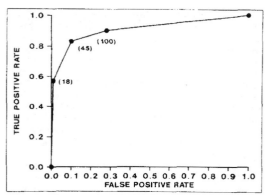

Figure 1. ROC curve for serum ferritin.

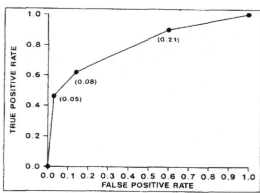

Figure 2. ROC curve for transferrin saturation.

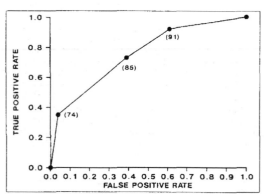

Figure 3. ROC curve for mean cell volume.

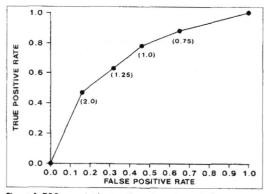

Figure 4. ROC curve for free erythrocyte protoporphyrin.

fied separately in the presentation of the results that follows.

A total of 1,334 patients over 65 years with anemia was identified. Of these, 259 proved eligible, participated in the study, and underwent bone marrow aspiration. Seventy-six participants were outpatients, and 183 were inpatients. Of the 259 bone marrow aspirates from the patients, 235 were interpretable (the quality being too poor in the others). The reasons for exclusion of anemic patients are presented in **Table I**. Most of the patients who recently received transfusions were postoperative patients, a large proportion of whom (at a hospital with a very busy orthopedic service) had undergone total hip replacement or had a recent hip fracture.

The mean age (± SD) of the participating patients was 79.7 ± 7.62 years; 119 (46%) were men. The mean hemoglobin level was 9.81 g/dL (± 1.39); 52.1% of the patients had a hemoglobin level less than 10.0 g/dL. A very wide variety of illnesses were not directly related to the anemia. Seventy-two patients had no medical diagnosis other than anemia (and its cause); 72 had one other diagnosis; 67 had two other diagnoses; 34 had three other diagnoses; and 14 had more than three other diagnoses. The most common medical diagnoses (aside from anemia), and the number of patients affected, were as follows: early dementia, 25; congestive heart failure, 25; chronic airflow limitation, 17; rheumatoid arthritis, 17; osteoarthritis, 14; pneumonia, 13.

The final diagnoses of anemia are presented in **Table II**. The weighted kappa-quantifying chance-corrected agreement for the 65 marrow aspirates that were interpreted by two hematologists was 0.84.

Figures 1 to 4 present the ROC curves for serum ferritin, transferrin saturation, MCV, and red cell protoporphyrin. Because, through administrative error and lost samples, all tests were not conducted in all subjects, the number of patients available for each analysis varied, and was sometimes less than 235. Examination of the ROC curves revealed that serum ferritin performed far better than any of the other tests. This was confirmed by the statistical analysis, which showed that the area under the ROC curves was 0.91, 0.79, 0.78, and 0.72 (respectively), for the four tests. Although the difference between the serum ferritin and the other three tests was statistically significant (p ≤0.001 in each case), any differences seen in the other four curves can easily be explained by chance (p ≥0.1).

Likelihood ratios for the four tests are presented in **Table III**. Consistent with the ROC curves, serum ferritin showed a far greater discriminative power than the other tests.

Likelihood ratios for RDW for distinguishing those with iron deficiency from those with anemia of chronic disease were examined. The likelihood ratios for RDW 0 to 15, 15 to 19, and greater than 19 were 0.39, 1.31, and 1.90, respectively. Ferritin proved a far more powerful predictor for differentiating iron deficiency from

TABLE III

Likelihood Ratios

Interval	Number Iron-Deficient	Number Not Iron-Deficient	Likelihood Ratio
Ferritin			
>100	8	108	0.13
>45 ≤ 100	7	27	0.46
>18 ≤ 45	23	13	3.12
≤18	47	2	41.47
Total	85	150	
Transferrin saturation			
>0.21	9	55	0.28
>0.8 ≤ 0.21	23	70	0.57
>0.05 ≤ 0.08	14	17	1.43
≤0.05	38	4	16.51
Total	84	146	
Mean cell volume			
>95	2	32	0.11
>91 − ≤ 95	5	26	0.34
>85 − ≤ 91	16	44	0.64
>74 − ≤ 85	32	42	1.35
≤74	30	6	8.82
Total	85	150	
Red cell protoporphyrin			
≥ 0 ≤ 0.75	10	53	0.34
>0.75 ≤ 0.1	8	28	0.51
>1 − ≤ 1.25	9	21	0.77
>1.25 ≤ 2	17	24	1.26
>2	40	24	2.98
Total	84	150	

TABLE IV

Likelihood Ratios from Logistic Regression Analysis

Interval	Number Iron-Deficient	Number Not Iron-Deficient	Likelihood Ratio
Ferritin			
Ferritin negative*†, transferrin saturation negative‡	13	126	0.18
Only ferritin positive	33	10	5.72
Ferritin positive, transferrin saturation positive	33	1	57.23
Total	79	137	

* Only four cases were serum ferritin-negative and transferrin saturation-positive.
† Cut-point for serum ferritin was 45 μg/L.
‡ Cut-point for transferrin saturation was 0.08.

TABLE V

Post-Test Probability of Iron Deficiency Given Varying Pre-Test Probabilities and Results of Serum Ferritin Determinations

	Pre-Test Probability			
	Low (5% − 20%)	Intermediate (40% − 60%)	High (80% − 95%)	Study Population (36%)
Serum ferritin result (μg/L)				
>100	0.6–3	8–16	34–71	7
45–100	2–10	24–41	39–90	21
18–45	14–44	68–82	93–98	64
<18	69–91	97–98	99–99.9	96

anemia of chronic disease, with likelihood ratios ranging from 0.05 to infinity. Finally, RDW added little to the predictive power of serum ferritin.

In the logistic regression model, ferritin was the best predictor of bone marrow iron stores. The only test that explained a statistically significant additional portion of the variance was the transferrin saturation. Using a cutoff of 45 μg/L for ferritin and 0.08 for transferrin saturation, likelihood ratios generated by using a combination of the tests are presented in **Table IV**. Little is gained by this model in comparison to serum ferritin: likelihood ratios greater than 1 are slightly higher, but the likelihood ratio less than 1 is not as low as the value obtained with a serum ferritin level of greater than 100 μg/L. Of patients with serum ferritin values of 18 to 100 μg/L, seven had transferrin saturation values of less than 0.05. All seven of these patients proved to be iron-deficient.

Other studies have reported elevated serum ferritin levels in patients with liver disease and inflammatory diseases, particularly rheumatoid arthritis [2,3,5,6,8,14,15]. Of the five patients with liver disease who were iron-deficient, three had serum ferritin values less than 18 μg/L. Of the six iron-deficient subjects with rheumatoid arthritis, five had a serum ferritin level less than 18 μg/L. Therefore, in our study, patients with liver disease or rheumatoid arthritis appeared to behave in a manner similar to that in the rest of the population. However, the numbers of patients with these conditions were insufficient to permit strong inference regarding the issue of differences among subgroups.

COMMENTS

Previous studies in younger subjects have consistently shown the usefulness of serum ferritin in the diagnosis of iron-deficiency anemia, and suggested that serum ferritin is more powerful than other blood tests [1–9]. Our results are consistent with these findings: in elderly patients with anemia, serum ferritin determination is by far the best test for diagnosis of iron deficiency. Other tests add only limited information in the diagnosis.

The MCV is ordinarily available with the complete blood count, and could thus influence the estimate of the probability of iron deficiency prior to ordering of other tests. However, in our population, even MCV values of less than 74 were not invariably associated with iron deficiency, and in many of the patients with iron deficiency the anemia was not microcytic. Only 6% of those with an MCV greater than 95 had iron deficiency; therefore, a very large MCV can be interpreted as virtually excluding iron deficiency.

The likelihood ratios for the possible ranges of results of serum ferritin determinations are presented in Table III. Previous studies in uncomplicated anemia have led to recommended cutoff points between normal and abnormal of 12 to 20 μg/L [1–9]. Using this approach, any value above 20 μg/L would be treated as a negative test result and as decreasing the likelihood of the patient having iron deficiency. In fact, in our population, ferritin values between 18 and 45 μg/L reflected an increase in the likelihood of iron deficiency (Table III), and the optimal cutoff in terms of maximizing accuracy was 45 μg/L (Figure 1). This result likely reflects the fact that serum ferritin levels in-

crease with age [13]. It may also reflect the high prevalence of chronic disease in the elderly, although only a
small proportion of our population had inflammatory
conditions thought to be associated with increased levels of serum ferritin.

Although these results might lead to the conclusion
that a higher cutoff for serum ferritin should be used
in the elderly, more information is to be gained by
using multiple cut-points. The clinical usefulness of
the likelihood ratios associated within different results of serum ferritin is illustrated in **Table V**. Table
V examines four different scenarios: patients with low
(5% to 20%), intermediate (40% to 60%), and high (80%
to 95%) pre-test probability or prevalence of iron deficiency as an explanation for their anemia, as well as
the population of the current study (in whom the prevalence of iron deficiency was 36%). The power of the
serum ferritin level is made evident by examining the
patients with intermediate probability, in whom the
post-test probability of iron deficiency decreases to 8%
to 16% if the serum ferritin level is greater than 100 μg/
L, while a result of less than 18 μg/L increases the
likelihood of iron deficiency to greater than 97%. Let
us assume a physician is willing to diagnose a patient
with a probability of 10% or less as not having iron-
deficiency anemia, and a patient with a probability of
90% or more as having iron deficiency, without performing a bone marrow examination. Under these circumstances, a serum ferritin value of greater than 45
μg/L will obviate the necessity of a bone marrow aspiration in all patients with low prior probability; and a
result of less than 18 μg/L in those with an intermediate prior probability, or less than 45 μg/L in those with
a high prior probability, secures the diagnosis of iron
deficiency.

The results depicted in the last column of Table IV
suggest that, for clinicians dealing with populations
similar to the one included in the present study, patients with values greater than 100 μg/L can be treated
as not having iron deficiency, patients with values of
less than 18 μg/L can be treated as having iron deficiency, and a bone marrow aspiration is necessary for
diagnosis in those with intermediate values. Using this
approach would lead to a diagnosis of iron deficiency
in 21% of the patients, and exclusion of iron deficiency
in 49%. Thus, bone marrow aspiration would be required in only 30%.

The present study has a number of strengths in
comparison to previous investigations of the usefulness of laboratory tests in the diagnosis of iron deficiency. The sample represents a group of consecutive
elderly patients presenting with anemia. We demonstrated the reproducibility of the interpretation of results of bone marrow aspiration, the procedure was
undertaken in all patients, and the findings were interpreted by a hematologist unaware of the results of the
laboratory investigations. We can therefore be confident of our conclusion that serum ferritin is the one
peripheral blood test useful in the diagnosis of iron-
deficiency anemia in the elderly; that the results

should be interpreted differently from serum ferritin
results in younger patients; and that when the information from the test is optimally utilized (by means of
multi-level likelihood ratios), the test is extremely
powerful in the diagnosis of iron-deficiency anemia.

ACKNOWLEDGMENT

We thank the following individuals for their help in data collection and preparation
of this manuscript: Dr. Anne Benger for help with interpretation of bone marrow
aspirates; and Sue Halcrow, Sandi Harper, Jenny Whyte, and Debbie Maddock for
help with data collection, data processing, and manuscript preparation.

REFERENCES

1. Beck JR, Gibbons AB, Cornwell G, et al: Multivariate approach to predictive
diagnosis of bone-marrow iron stores. Am J Clin Pathol 1979; 70: S665–S670.
2. Sheehan RG, Newton MJ, Frenkel EP: Evaluation of a packaged kit assay of
serum ferritin and application to clinical diagnosis of selected anemias. Am J Clin
Pathol 1978; 70: 79–84.
3. Krause JR, Stoic V: Serum ferritin and bone marrow biopsy iron stores. Am J Clin
Pathol 1980; 74: S461–S464.
4. Ali MAM, Luxton AW, Walker WHC: Serum ferritin concentration and bone marrow iron stores: a prospective study. Can Med Assoc J 1978; 118: 945–946.
5. Mazza J, Barr RM, McDonald JWD, Valberg LS: Usefulness of the serum ferritin
concentration in the detection of iron deficiency in a general hospital. Can Med
Assoc J 1978; 119: 884–886.
6. Sorbie J, Valberg LS, Corbett WEN, Ludwig J: Serum ferritin, cobalt excretion
and body iron status. Can Med Assoc J 1975; 112: 1173–1178.
7. Addison GM, Beamish MR, Hales CN, et al: An immunoradiometric assay for
ferritin in the serum of normal subjects and patients with iron deficiency and iron
overload. J Clin Pathol 1972; 25: 326–329.
8. Lipschitz DA, Cook JD, Finch CA: A clinical evaluation of serum ferritin as an
index of iron stores. N Engl J Med 1974; 290: 1213–1216.
9. Walsh JR, Fredrickson M: Serum ferritin, free erythrocyte protoporphyrin, and
urinary iron excretion in patients with iron disorders. Am J Med Sci 1977; 273:
293–300.
10. Pirie R: The influence of age upon serum iron in normal subjects. J Clin Pathol
1952; 5: 10–15.
11. Yip R, Johnson C, Dallman PR: Age-related changes in laboratory values used in
the diagnosis of anemia and iron deficiency. Am J Clin Nutr 1984; 39: 427–436.
12. Powell DEB, Thomas JH: The iron binding capacity of serum in elderly hospital
patients. Gerontol Clin (Basel) 1969; 11: 36–47.
13. Loria A, Hershko C, Konij N: Serum ferritin in an elderly population. J Gerontol
1979; 34: 521–525.
14. Nelson R, Chawla M, Connolly P, Laporte J: Ferritin as an index of bone marrow
iron stores. South Med J 1978; 71: 1482–1484.
15. Bentley DP, Williams P: Serum ferritin concentration as an index of storage iron
in rheumatoid arthritis. J Clin Pathol 1974; 27: 786–788.
16. Patterson C, Turpie ID, Benger AM: Assessment of iron stores in anemic geriatric patients. J Am Geriatr Soc 1985; 33: 746–767.
17. Awad MO, Berford AV, Grindulis KA, et al: Factors affecting the serum iron-
binding capacity in the elderly. Gerontology 1982; 28: 125–131.
18. Lynch SR, Finch CA, Monsen ER, et al: Iron status of elderly Americans. Am J
Clin Nutr 1982; 36: 1032–1045.
19. Department of Clinical Epidemiology and Biostatistics, McMaster University:
Interpretation of diagnostic data: how to do it with simple maths. Can Med Assoc J
1983; 129: 22–29.
20. International Committee for Standardization in Haematology: The measurement of total iron and unsaturated iron binding capacity in serum. Br J Haematol
1978; 38: 281–287.
21. Luxton AW, Walker WHC, Gauldie J, Ali MAM, Pelletier C: A radioimmunoassay
for serum ferritin. Clin Chem 1977; 23: 683–689.
22. Piomelli S, Young P, Gay G: A micro method for free erythrocyte protoporphyrin: the FEP test. J Lab Clin Med 1973; 81: 932–940.
23. Dacie SV, Lewis SM: Practical hematology, 6th ed. New York: Churchill Livingstone, 1984: 107–109.
24. Hanley JA, McNeil BJ: The meaning and use of the area under a receiver
operating characteristic (ROC) curve. Radiology 1982; 143: 29–36.
25. Hanley JA, McNeil BJ: A method of comparing the areas under receiver operating characteristic curves derived from the same cases. Radiology 1983; 148: 839–
843.

March 1990 The American Journal of Medicine Volume 88 209

Citation:

Are the results of this diagnostic study valid?

Was there an independent, blind comparison with a reference ('gold') standard of diagnosis?

Was the diagnostic test evaluated in an appropriate spectrum of patients (like those in whom it would be used in practice)?

Was the reference standard applied regardless of the diagnostic test result?

Are the valid results of this diagnostic study important?

SAMPLE CALCULATIONS (*see* p120 of *Evidence-based Medicine*)

		Target disorder (iron deficiency anaemia)		Totals
		Present	**Absent**	
Diagnostic test result	Positive (<65 mmol/L)	731 a	270 b	a+b 1001
(serum ferritin)	Negative (≥65 mmol/L)	78 c	1500 d	c+d 1578
	Totals	809 a+c	1770 b+d	a+b+c+d 2579

Sensitivity = a/(a+c) = 731/809 = 90%

Specificity = d/(b+d) = 1500/1770 = 85%

Likelihood Ratio for a positive test result = LR+ = sens/(1 – spec) = 90%/15% = 6

Likelihood Ratio for a negative test result = LR– = (1–sens)/spec = 10%/85% = 0.12

Positive Predictive Value = a/(a+b) = 731/1001 = 73%

Negative Predictive Value = d/(c+d) = 1500/1578 = 95%

Pre-test Probability (prevalence) = (a+c)/(a+b+c+d) = 809/2579 = 32%

Pre-test-odds = prevalence/(1 – prevalence) = 31%/69% = 0.45

Post-test odds = Pre-test odds x Likelihood Ratio

Post-test Probability = Post-test odds/(Post-test odds + 1)

Are the valid results of this diagnostic study important?

YOUR CALCULATIONS

		Target Disorder		Totals
		Present	**Absent**	
Diagnostic test result	Positive	a	b	a+b
	Negative	c	d	c+d
	Totals	a+c	b+d	a+b+c+d

Sensitivity = a/(a+c) =   Specificity = d/(b+d) =

Likelihood Ratio for a positive test result = LR+ = sens/(1–spec) =

Likelihood Ratio for a negative test result = LR– = (1-sens)/spec =

Positive Predictive Value = a/(a+b) =   Negative Predictive Value = d/(c+d) =

Pre-test Probability (prevalence) = (a+c)/(a+b+c+d) =

Pre-test-odds = prevalence/(1–prevalence) =

Post-test odds = Pre-test odds x Likelihood Ratio =

Post-test Probability = Post-test odds/(Post-test odds + 1) =

Can you apply this valid, important evidence about a diagnostic test in caring for your patient?

Is the diagnostic test available, affordable, accurate, and precise in your setting?

Can you generate a clinically sensible estimate of your patient's pre-test probability (from practice data, personal experience, the report itself, or clinical speculation).

Will the resulting post-test probabilities affect your management and help your patient? (Could it move you across a test-treatment threshold? Would your patient be a willing partner in carrying it out?)

Would the consequences of the test help your patient?

Additional notes

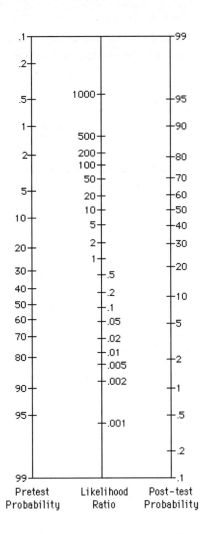

Pretest Probability — Likelihood Ratio — Post-test Probability

Anchor a straight-edge along the left edge of the nomogram at your patient's pre-test probability and pivot it until it intersects the likelihood ratio for your patent's diagnostic test result. It will intersect the right edge of the nomogram at your patient's post-test probability. Test 1: for a likelihood ratio of 1, pre-test and post-test probabilities should be identical. Test 2: for a pre-test probability of 30% and a likelihood ratio of 5, the post-test probability is just under 70%.

Adapted from Fagan TJ (1975) Nomogram for Bayes' theorem. *N Engl J Med.* **293**: 257.

Citation: Guyatt GH, Patterson C, Ali M, Singer J, *et al.* (1990) Diagnosis of iron-deficiency anemia in the elderly. *Am J Med.* **88**: 205–9

Are the results of this diagnostic study valid?

Was there an independent, blind comparison with a reference ('gold') standard of diagnosis?	**Yes, they underwent bone-marrow aspirations.**
Was the diagnostic test evaluated in an appropriate spectrum of patients (like those in whom it would be used in practice)?	**Yes.**
Was the reference standard applied regardless of the diagnostic test result?	**Yes.**

Are the valid results of this diagnostic study important?

Ferritin	Iron deficiency	No iron deficiency	Likelihood ratio
≤45	70/85	15/150	8.2
>45≤100	7/85	27/150	0.44
>100	8/85	108/150	0.13
Totals	85	150	

- **For pre-test probabilities in the 30–70% range, a ferritin ≤45 would be very helpful, yielding post-test probabilities of 78–95% (in the latter case, a SpPin[1]).**

- **In that same pre-test probability range, a ferritin >100 would yield post-test probabilities of 5–23% (in the former case, a SnNou[2]).**

- **So it can give quite important results.**

[1] When a diagnostic test has a very high **Sp**ecificity, a **P**ositive result Rules-**In** the diagnosis.

[2] When a diagnostic test has a very high **Se**nsitivity, a **N**egative result Rules-**Out** the diagnosis.

Can you apply this valid, important evidence about a diagnostic test in caring for your patient?

Is the diagnostic test available, affordable, accurate, and precise in your setting?	**Needs to be assessed in each setting.**
Can you generate a clinically sensible estimate of your patient's pre-test probability (from practice data, personal experience, the report itself, or clinical speculation)?	**Approximately 30%.**
Will the resulting post-test probabilities affect your management and help your patient? (Could it move you across a test-treatment threshold? Would your patient be a willing partner in carrying it out?)	**Her result of 40 brings her post-test probability to 78%, certainly high enough for you to want to investigate her for causes of anaemia (GI loss, etc.).**
Would the consequences of the test help your patient?	**Yes, if it led to a reversible cause. But this would have to be weighed against early detection of an untreatable cause, e.g. cancer, that would simply take away 'healthy' time. The options would need to be discussed with your patient.**

Additional notes

1 An excellent overview of 55 studies of lab tests for Fe-deficient anaemia: Guyatt *et al.* (1992) *J Gen Intern Med.* **7**: 145–53 (with a correction on page 423).

A LIKELIHOOD RATIO NOMOGRAM

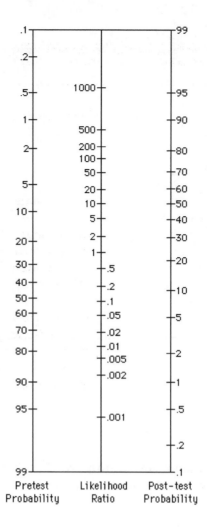

Pretest Probability	Likelihood Ratio	Post-test Probability

Anchor a straight-edge along the left edge of the nomogram at your patient's pre-test probability and pivot it until it intersects the likelihood ratio for your patent's diagnostic test result. It will intersect the right edge of the nomogram at your patient's post-test probability. Test 1: for a likelihood ratio of 1, pre-test and post-test probabilities should be identical. Test 2: for a pre-test probability of 30% and a likelihood ratio of 5, the post-test probability is just under 70%.

Adapted from Fagan TJ (1975) Nomogram for Bayes' theorem. *N Engl J Med.* **293:** 257.

Clinical Bottom Line

In community-dwelling elderly medical patients in whom iron deficiency anaemia is suspected, serum ferritin is a valid, precise diagnostic test.

Citation

Guyatt GH, Patterson C, Ali M *et al.* (1990) Diagnosis of iron-deficiency anemia in the elderly. *Am J Med* **88:** 205–9.

Clinical Question

In a patient with anaemia can a low serum ferritin be used to diagnose iron deficiency anaemia in the elderly?

Search Terms

'ferritin' and 'sensitivity and specificity' in MEDLINE.

The Study

1 Gold Standard – bone marrow aspiration.

2 Study setting – consecutive pts over the age of 65 who were admitted with anaemia to a university-affiliated hospital in Canada.

The Evidence

Ferritin	Iron deficiency	No iron deficiency	Likelihood ratio
≤45	70/85	15/150	8.2
>45≤100	7/85	27/150	0.44
>100	8/85	108/150	0.13
Totals	85	150	

Comments

1 Excluded pts from institutions and pts who were 'too ill' or had 'severe dementia' although these were not defined.

2 Weighted kappa for bone marrow interpretation by 2 haematologists was 0.84.

3 Low values can SpPin, and high values can SnNout.

4 Also see the meta-analysis in *J Gen Intern Med* 1992; **7:** 145–53 (with a correction on page 423).

DIAGNOSIS OF IRON DEFICIENCY ANEMIA IN THE ELDERLY

Appraised by Sharon Straus: Nov 1996.
Expiry date: 2000.

SOURCES OF EVIDENCE FOR EVIDENCE-BASED MEDICINE

Title	Medium	Content type	Advantages	Disadvantages
Best Evidence on Disk (American College of Physicians & BMJ Publications Group)	CD-ROM or diskette (cumulated contents of two paper journals: *ACP Journal Club* and *Evidence-based Medicine*.) Updated every year.	Structured abstracts of articles from selected journals in internal medicine, general practice, obstetrics and gynaecology, paediatrics, psychiatry, and surgery. Articles must meet strict quality criteria; each abstract (evidence) accompanied by a commentary (clinical expertise).	High quality evidence with commentary; easy to search; high specificity (not much time wasted with irrelevant material).	Incomplete coverage of literature: low sensitivity.

WHEN TO USE IT: *As your first port of call for the specialities it covers.*

Title	Medium	Content type	Advantages	Disadvantages
Cochrane Library	CD-ROM or diskette or Internet	Superb evidence about therapy & prevention; systematic reviews; abstracts of overviews of effectiveness.	Highest quality evidence we'll ever have on the effectiveness of health care.	Not yet many Cochrane reviews; necessarily omits the newest treatments.

WHEN TO USE IT: *As your best port of call for therapy.*

Title	Medium	Content type	Advantages	Disadvantages
MEDLINE (US National Library of Medicine)	Networked CD-ROM systems; on-line vendors. (SilverPlatter [WinSPIRS] Ovid, etc.)	Bibliographic records, with abstract and MeSH terms. Full-text services starting to appear.	Exhaustiveness; flexibility of searching; journal coverage; currency (on-line versions); widespread availability and support (lots of people can help you!)	Have to do your own quality filtering; putting together good searches is difficult; gaps in coverage (medical, geographical and linguistic).

WHEN TO USE IT: *When you need to be sure you've got everything and have time to search properly.*

Title	Medium	Content type	Advantages	Disadvantages
World-Wide Web (WWW)	Internet (via browser programs such as Netscape, MS Internet Explorer, Mosaic, Yahoo, Lynx, etc.)	Everything: from LRs to NNTs; electronic journals (e.g. Bandolier) & journal clubs; software tools; CATs; teaching materials; searching tips; events and conferences; etc.	Some sites are excellent, with high-quality pre-filtered evidence; some good, free software; boundless possibilities; can be updated instantly.	Variable levels of quality control; poor sensitivity and specificity; access from NHS networks can be problematic; can be slow to download.

WHEN TO USE IT: *Find good sites and check them regularly for updates.*

Recommended sites:	CEBM	http://cebm.jr2.ox.ac.uk/	CATs, NNTs, LRs, etc., teaching materials, announcements, links to other sites.	
	SCHARR / AurACLE	http://www.shef.ac.uk/~scharr/ir/netting.html	Evidence-based information seeking, links to other sites.	
	Bandolier	http://www.jr2.ox.ac.uk/Bandolier/	An electronic version (including back issues) of the EBM journal *Bandolier*.	
WWW search services	General comment on Web searching	Allow you to type in keywords and search an index of WWW pages.	Tens of millions of pages are indexed and can be accessed directly. Searching is crude and hits displayed in an order which is not always appropriate.	
Typical specific services:	Yahoo!	http://www.yahoo.com	More selective than most search sites, though this may not coincide with your needs!	
	AltaVista	http://www.altavista.com	Seems to be the most exhaustive, with best searching engine.	

WHEN TO USE IT: *To find very specific information from the Web or starting points for browsing.*

PART

 A

Critical appraisal of a clinical article about prognosis

You see a 70-year old man in an outpatient clinical three months after he has been discharged from your service with an ischaemic (presumed thrombotic) stroke. He is in sinus rhythm, has mild residual left-sided weakness but is otherwise well. His only medication is aspirin and he has no allergies. He recently saw an article on the BMJ website describing the risk of seizure after a stroke and is concerned that this will happen to him. Together you form the question: 'In patients with a history of stroke, what is the risk of seizure within the first year?'

You search MEDLINE using the terms 'stroke' and 'seizure' and find the article he was referring to: *BMJ* (1997) **315:** 1582–7.

Read the article and decide:
1   Is this evidence about prognosis valid?
2   Is this valid evidence about prognosis important?
3   Can you apply this valid and important evidence about prognosis in caring for your patient?

If you want to read some strategies for answering these sorts of questions, you could have a look at pp 85–90, 129–32 and 164–5 in *Evidence-based Medicine.*

Prognosis and introduction to the CATMaker software

PART

B

Introduction to the CATMaker software (optional)

We will give you a copy of the CATMaker and show you how to use it to generate and save your own one-page 'Critically Appraised Topic (CAT)' from an article about therapy. The advantages of the CATMaker include its ability to calculate for you the clinically useful measures of the effects of therapy and their confidence intervals, and to save your critical appraisal for printing, sharing and storage.

Now would be a good time to start searching on potential topics for your presentations in Sessions 6 and 7!

Epileptic seizures after a first stroke: the Oxfordshire community stroke project

John Burn, Martin Dennis, John Bamford, Peter Sandercock, Derick Wade, Charles Warlow

Rehabilitation
Research Unit,
Southampton
General Hospital,
Southampton
SO9 4XY
John Burn,
*consultant in
rehabilitation
medicine*

continued over

BMJ 1997;315:1582–7

Abstract

Objective: To describe the immediate and long term risk of epileptic seizures after a first ever stroke.

Design: Cohort study following up stroke survivors for 2 to 6.5 years; comparison with age specific incidence rates of epileptic seizures in the general population.

Setting: Community based stroke register.

Subjects: 675 patients with a first stroke, followed up for a minimum of 2 years.

Main outcome measures: Occurrence of single and recurrent seizures.

Results: 52 patients had one or more post stroke seizures; in 25 the seizures were recurrent. The 5 year actuarial risk of a post stroke seizure in survivors (excluding 19 patients with a history of epilepsy and 3 patients in whom the seizure occurred shortly before death from another cause) was 11.5% (95% confidence interval 4.8% to 18.2%). The relative risk of seizures, in comparison with the general population, was estimated at 35.2 in the first year after stroke and 19.0 in year 2. The risk of seizures was increased in survivors of subarachnoid and intracerebral haemorrhage (hazard ratio for intracranial haemorrhage v cerebral infarction 10.2 (3.7 to 27.9)). The risk of seizures after ischaemic stroke was substantial only in patients presenting with severe strokes due to total anterior circulation infarction. Only 9 of 295 patients (3%) independent one month after stroke suffered a seizure between 1 month and 5 years (actuarial risk 4.2% (0.1% to 8.3%)).

Conclusion: Stroke patients have about an 11.5% risk of single or recurrent seizures in the first 5 years after a stroke. Patients with more severe strokes or haemorrhagic strokes are at higher risk.

Introduction

Cerebrovascular disease is an important cause of epilepsy,[1] particularly in elderly people.[2] When seizures complicate a clinical stroke they have a devastating effect on morale and further impair an already compromised quality of life. Precise estimates of the risk of developing epilepsy would be helpful not only to patients but also to those who give advice on returning to work or driving. Data from hospital based studies may give falsely high estimates of risk since patients with severe strokes, or strokes presenting with seizures, may be more likely to be admitted to hospital.[3] In this study we had three aims: to describe the immediate and long term risk of epileptic seizures after a first stroke among patients in a community stroke register; to analyse the occurrence of seizures in relation to the pathological and clinical subtype of first stroke; and to compare the risk of a first epileptic seizure in these stroke patients with the risk in the general population.

Method

The cohort

The Oxfordshire community stroke project registered 675 patients with a first stroke, 357 (53%) women and 318 (47%) men, from a study population of about 105 000 over 4 years. Patients of all ages were included: 163 (24%) were under 65 years, 195 (29%) 65-74 years, 228 (34%) 75-84 years, and 89 (13%) over 84 years (mean age 72.2 years). Patients were recruited between 1981 and 1986 and were followed up until 1988, when the project finished (minimum follow up 2 years). The methods used to identify and assess cases have been described elsewhere.[4 5] A total of 545 patients (81%) had cerebral infarction, 66 (10%) primary intracerebral haemorrhage, and 33 (5%) subarachnoid haemorrhage. In 31 (4%) cases the type of stroke could not be determined.

Ten patients had intracranial operations for aneurysm, and five of these patients received prophylactic phenytoin for 18 months to 2 years. Prophylactic anticonvulsant treatment was not offered to any other patients. One patient with primary intracerebral haemorrhage (not complicated by seizures) had intracranial surgery.

All but two of the 545 patients with cerebral infarction could be classified into subtypes according to their clinical presentation[6]: 92 patients had total anterior circulation infarction (cortical and subcortical ischaemia likely to be due to occlusion of the main stem of the middle cerebral artery or of the internal carotid artery); 185 patients had partial anterior circulation infarction (predominantly cortical ischaemia likely to be due to occlusion of a branch of the middle cerebral or anterior cerebral artery); 137 patients had lacunar infarction (a lacunar syndrome likely to be due to intracerebral small vessel occlusion[7]); and 129 patients had posterior circulation infarction (ischaemia in the brainstem, cerebellum or occipital cortex likely to be due to either small or large vessel occlusion).

Follow up

Survivors were interviewed by a study nurse at 1 month, 6 months, 12 months, and then annually around the anniversary of their first stroke. At each follow up the nurse asked the patient and caregivers specifically about whether any possible seizure had occurred. As a check the nurse also reviewed the records kept by the primary healthcare team. Patients with suspected seizures were reassessed clinically by the study neurologist. Long term survivors were visited at the close of the study by one of the study neurologists (JPSB), and all available information about possible seizures was reviewed again with the patient. The hospital and primary care records of patients who died before this final visit were reviewed by one of the study neurologists (JPSB), and data relating to possible seizures were discussed at regular consensus meetings of the study team. Generalised seizures were diagnosed with reference to statements of witnesses. Focal seizures were distinguished clinically from clonus, spasms, and recurrent strokes.[8 9] Electroencephalograms were not routinely performed. Each visit included an assessment of functional ability using the Oxford handicap scale[10]; in this report patients in grades 0-2 were described as independent and patients in grades 3-5 as dependent.

The Oxfordshire community stroke project followed up every patient for 2 years or until death. Patients recruited earlier in the study were followed for longer, and no patient was lost to follow up. Seventeen patients died on day 1, 129 by 30 days, 208 by 1 year, and 254 by 2 years. A total of 421 patients were followed up at 2 years, 274 were seen at 3 years, 182 at 4 years, and 92 at 5 years; 324 patients survived to a final examination by a study neurologist between August 1987 and November 1988.

Classification of seizures

Onset seizures were defined as occurring within 24 hours of the onset of stroke. This definition (see appendix) is based on that used in a population based study of acute seizures after head injury.[11] Seizures occurring later were classified as post stroke seizures, except in two cases where evolution of stroke was prolonged.

Comparison with the general population

The incidence of post stroke seizures was compared with the estimated rate of epileptic seizures in the general population, using data from the VAMP research bank, a large British primary care database.[12 13] Eighty two practices had sent in data on the medical and prescribing history of 369 819 patients. The data were checked for completeness and internal consistency,[13] and practices supplying unreliable data were excluded.

Statistical methods

Actuarial analysis was used for cohort data involving the follow up of patients for varying lengths of time. Kaplan-Meier survival curves were constructed in which patients who died or were no longer being followed up (after 2 years) were censored. The occurrence of a post stroke seizure qualified as an end point, and these were graphically represented as a cumulative seizure rate. Different pathological types, age stratifications, and clinical subtypes of stroke were compared by using the log rank method.[14] The incidence of epileptic seizures was compared between stroke survivors and the general population and expressed as a ratio of the observed to the expected frequency with confidence intervals calculated from the Poisson distribution.[15] Calculations were made for year 1 and year 2 separately; there were insufficient events to continue this comparison in years 3-5. Confidence intervals of small samples were calculated by using an exact test.[15]

Department of Clinical Neurosciences, Western General Hospital, Edinburgh EH4 2XU
Martin Dennis, *senior lecturer in stroke medicine*
Peter Sandercock, *reader in medical neurology*
Charles Warlow, *professor of medical neurology*

Department of Neurology, St James's University Hospital, Leeds LS9 7TF
John Bamford, *consultant neurologist*

Rivermead Rehabilitation Centre, Oxford OX1 4XD
Derick Wade, *consultant neurologist*

Correspondence to: Dr Burn rehab@soton.ac.uk

Table 1 Frequency of onset seizures and development of post stroke seizures by type of first stroke

Type of first stroke	No (%; 95% CI) of patients with onset seizures	Number (%) of patients with onset seizures who developed post stroke seizures
Cerebral infarction (n=545)	10 (2; 0.9 to 3.4)	4 (40)
Primary intracerebral haemorrhage (n=66)	2 (3; 0.4 to 10.5)	1 (50)
Subarachnoid haemorrhage (n=33)	2 (6; 0.7 to 20.2)	0
Unknown (n=31)	0 (0; 0 to 11.2)	0
Total (n=675)	14 (2; 1.1 to 3.5)	5 (36)

Table 2 Number (% of cohort; 95% confidence interval) of patients with single and recurrent seizures after first stroke (four patients who had seizures within a few hours of death as part of a terminal illness, or seizures that started before the stroke, were excluded)

Classification of first stroke	Single post stroke seizure	Recurrent post stroke seizures	Total
Cerebral infarction (n=545):	17 (3)	18 (3)	35 (6; 4 to 9)
Total anterior circulation infarction (n=92)	5 (5)	10 (11)	15 (16)
Partial anterior circulation infarction (n=185)	5 (3)	3 (2)	8 (4)
Lacunar infarction (n=137)	3 (2)	2 (1)	5 (3)
Posterior circulation infarction (n=129)	4 (3)	3 (2)	7 (5)
Primary intracerebral haemorrhage (n=66)	3 (5)	4 (6)	7 (11; 3 to 18)
Subarachnoid haemorrhage (n=33)	3 (9)	3 (9)	6 (18; 5 to 31)
Unknown (n=31)	0	0	0
Total (n=675)	23 (3)	25 (4)	48 (7; 6 to 9)

Table 3 Cumulative actuarial risks (95% confidence intervals) of experiencing a seizure after stroke by type of first stroke (19 patients with a history of prestroke seizures were excluded)

Time after stroke	Cerebral infarction	Primary intracerebral haemorrhage	Subarachnoid haemorrhage	Total
1 year	4.2 (2.2 to 6.2)	19.9 (1.5 to 38.3)	22.0 (2.6 to 41.8)	5.7 (3.5 to 7.9)
2 years	6.7 (4.1 to 9.3)	19.9 (1.5 to 38.3)	27.8 (5.3 to 50.7)	8.2 (5.4 to 11.0)
3 years	7.4 (4.0 to 10.8)	26.1 (2.2 to 50.0)	34.3 (8.0 to 62.0)	9.5 (5.8 to 13.2)
4 years	8.6 (4.5 to 12.7)	26.1 (1.3 to 50.9)	34.3 (2.0 to 68.1)	10.5 (6.0 to 15.0)
5 years	9.7 (3.7 to 15.7)	26.1 (0 to 54.8)	34.3 (0 to 100)	11.5 (4.8 to 18.2)

Results

Seizures preceding stroke

Nineteen of the 675 patients (3%) registered with the Oxfordshire community stroke project gave a history of one or more seizures before their first stroke or had documentation of past seizures in their medical record. In one patient the seizures were secondary to a craniotomy for a benign tumour; in one they occurred in the context of eclampsia; and in two they were related to alcohol abuse. The remaining seizures were considered idiopathic, and some may have been caused by otherwise asymptomatic cerebrovascular disease. Eleven of the 19 patients had had a seizure in the year before the stroke: in seven this was a first seizure, and four of these seven patients had partial motor seizures in the same limb as was subsequently affected by the stroke.

Seizures at the onset of the first stroke

Fourteen patients (2%) had an onset seizure, none of whom had a previous history of seizures. In seven the seizure was generalised, in six it was a simple partial seizure, and in one it was a complex partial seizure.

The occurrence of an onset seizure was not, in this cohort, associated with a worse outcome. The 30 day case fatality rate of patients with onset seizures was not raised. Two patients (14%) with onset seizures died compared with 127 of the 661 without onset seizures

(19.2%, 95% confidence interval 16.2% to 22.2%). There was also no suggestion that patients with onset seizures had a worse functional prognosis. Three of ten previously independent patients with onset seizures were dependent at one month compared with 179 of those without onset seizures (38.3%, 33.9% to 42.7%).

The occurrence of an onset seizure was, however, associated with an increased risk of having further seizures. Five (36%) of the 14 patients with onset seizures went on to have one or more post stroke seizures compared with 43 (6.9%) of 625 patients who survived the first day without a history of pre-stroke or onset seizures (odds ratio 7.52, 2.46 to 22.98).

Patients with subarachnoid haemorrhage had an excess of onset seizures but this was not statistically significant. Four (4%) of the 99 patients with intracranial haemorrhage had an onset seizure compared with 10 (1.8%) of the 545 patients with cerebral infarction (odds ratio 2.25, 0.69 to 7.33) (table 1).

Post stroke seizures

Fifty two (8%) of 658 patients who survived the first day had one or more post stroke seizures. Three patients had their first seizure only a few hours before death as part of the terminal illness and one patient had had seizures before the stroke. Most analyses were restricted to the remaining 48 patients. Twenty three patients had only a single post stroke seizure; 25 patients had recurrent post stroke seizures as defined in the appendix (table 2), but these generally occurred infrequently; only eight patients had more than one seizure a month over a period of two months or more. Only two of the five patients who had previously had an onset seizure went on to develop recurrent seizures.

Twenty four (50%) of the 48 patients were treated with anticonvulsant drugs; six of these had had only one post stroke seizure. Forty (83%) patients had at least one generalised seizure. Partial seizures occurring alone were less common than at the onset of the stroke.

Risk of post stroke seizure

A Kaplan-Meier survival curve was constructed in which the occurrence of a first post stroke seizure was recorded as an end point and deaths were censored (table 3, fig 1). Patients with a history of epilepsy before the stroke (n = 19) or who died in the first day after the stroke (n = 17) were excluded from these analyses. The probability of having a post stroke seizure was 5.7% (3.5% to 7.9%) within the first year and 11.5% (4.8% to 18.2%) within 5 years. The incremental risk averaged about 1.5% a year after the first 12 months. Five of the 10 patients who had a first seizure more than 2 years after the stroke had had another stroke more recently, and two had taken prophylactic phenytoin for two years after a subarachnoid haemorrhage.

The probability of a post stroke seizure was higher among patients aged over 84 years (observed/expected 2.0) but there was no significant trend on log rank analysis for an increasing risk with age ($\chi^2 = 0.91$, df = 1, P > 0.25). Subsequent analyses were not adjusted for age.

Patients who had had a haemorrhagic first stroke were more at risk of post stroke seizures than patients who had cerebral infarction (hazard ratio 10.2, 3.7 to 27.9) (table 3; fig 2). However, the lower risk after cerebral infarction concealed a significant hetero-

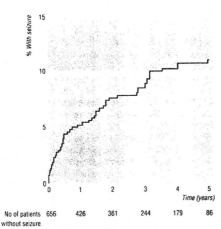

No of patients 656   426   361   244   179   86
without seizure

Fig 1 Kaplan-Meier estimate of the risk of post stroke seizures after first stroke: bars indicate 95% confidence intervals. Patients with a history of prestroke seizures (n=19) were excluded and deaths censored. Number of patients still being followed up at 1-5 years who had not had a seizure are indicated. Six of the 92 patients still being followed up at 5 years had had a previous seizure

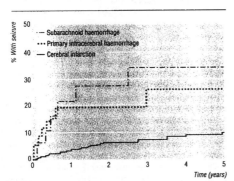

Fig 2 Kaplan-Meier estimate of post stroke seizures subdivided by type of stroke

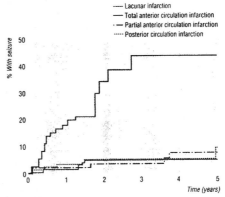

Fig 3 Kaplan-Meier estimates of post stroke seizures after cerebral infarction, subdivided by clinical subtype

geneity between different subtypes ($\chi^2 = 34.0$, df = 3, P < 0.001) (table 2; fig 3).

Survivors of total anterior circulation infarction had a markedly increased risk of post stroke seizures when compared with the survivors of other subtypes of cerebral infarction.

The good prognosis for survivors of partial anterior circulation infarction, lacunar infarction, and posterior circulation infarction was reflected in the low probability of future post stroke seizures among independent stroke survivors (those with Oxford handicap scale score 0-2). A further Kaplan-Meier curve restricted to patients alive and independent at 1 month revealed an incremental risk of suffering a post stroke seizure of about 0.9% a year and an actuarial risk at 5 years of 4.2% (0.1% to 8.3%). If only survivors independent at 6 months were included the 5 year actuarial risk was 2.7% (0 to 6.0%).

Comparison with the general population

Forty eight patients had at least one post stroke seizure recorded in a total follow up period (for patients with-

out a history of epilepsy) of 1641 patient years—an incidence of 29.3 patients developing post stroke seizures per 1000 patient years, or 23.5 per 1000 patient years when patients with intracerebral infarction, subarachnoid haemorrhage, or unknown pathology were excluded. This incidence was compared year by year for the first 2 years after stroke with the age specific incidence in the general population, as recorded by the VAMP research data bank over the 12 months between 1 February 1989 and 31 January 1990. Stroke survivors had a 35-fold increased risk of seizures in the first year (table 4). The increase in risk was particularly evident for patients under 65 years.

Discussion

An earlier, community based study of seizures after stroke reported that 9.5% of 518 survivors suffered a seizure 2-5 years after stroke, but no mention was made of subjects who were not followed up or who had died before the assessment.[16] Such problems can be addressed by an actuarial analysis which censors patients who die or who are lost to follow up. This method of analysis has been used in hospital based studies of epilepsy after stroke in New York[17] and Sweden[18] and in a population based study of seizures after cerebral infarction in Rochester, Minnesota.[19] The 5% risk of developing recurrent seizures by 5 years after the stroke found in the Swedish study[18] is similar to the risk observed in the Oxfordshire community stroke project (5.4%, 0.3% to 10.5%). The New York study reported a 19% risk of single or recurrent seizures by six years after an ischaemic stroke[17]; much higher than the risk we observed after cerebral infarction. This study, reported only in abstract, was retrospective and patients with post stroke seizures may have been preferentially followed up. An admission bias towards more patients with severe strokes[20] may also have raised the rate of seizures.

Seizures before stroke

The identification of seizures occurring shortly before the stroke offers support for the concept of vascular precursor epilepsy.[21] Eleven (2%) patients in the Oxfordshire study had a seizure in the year before the

BMJ VOLUME 315   13 DECEMBER 1997

stroke. This was three times the number expected in the general population.[22] A case-control study has shown an eightfold increased risk of epilepsy preceding stroke but was confounded by admission bias and the use of elective surgical admissions as controls,[23 24] and a study of patients investigated with computed tomography at the time of their first clinical stroke has confirmed evidence of preceding asymptomatic cerebral infarctions in 11% of patients; half of these involved the cerebral cortex.[25] Prestroke seizures could have arisen from such areas.

Seizures at onset of stroke

The Oxfordshire community stroke project recorded a lower rate of onset seizures than other studies which used a similar definition but in which a selection bias may have raised the rate.[26–28] These studies, which found rates in excess of 4%, were restricted to patients admitted to hospital, and the much quoted study by Aring and Merritt included only cases coming to necropsy.[28] This overrepresentation of fatal cases would have led to an excess of haemorrhagic strokes that were both epileptogenic and fatal.

A more representative hospital series of 1000 consecutive patients admitted to an Australian hospital with acute stroke identified 4.4% of patients with onset seizures and 3.5% with seizures after cerebral infarction.[29] The incidence among patients in the Oxfordshire study was lower, but the Australian series used an extended definition of onset seizures, including events that occurred up to 2 weeks from stroke onset. With the same definition, four more Oxfordshire patients with ischaemic stroke would be included and the incidence of onset seizures after cer-

ebral infarction would rise to 2.7% (1.5% to 3.9%), similar to the Australian result.

In the population based study from Rochester 4.8% of patients had an onset seizure within 24 hours of cerebral infarction,[19] a higher rate than in the Oxfordshire study. The Rochester series may have included patients with haemorrhagic lesions as these subjects had sustained their first stroke between 1960 and 1969, before the use of computed tomography scanning. A more recent series of 1195 hospital patients with both ischaemic and haemorrhagic stroke, which used the same two week definition of onset seizures, reported an incidence of 4.2%.[30] The occurrence of onset seizures in this study was associated, in a multiple regression analysis, with severity of the initial stroke, but the occurrence of an onset seizure did not in this study, or in the Oxfordshire study, necessarily indicate a worse outcome.

Onset seizures after stroke had features in common with acute seizures occurring after traumatic brain injury: the frequency of seizures occurring within 24 hours of the event was similar[11 31]: onset seizures were more often partial[31–33]; and the occurrence of an onset seizure increased the risk of later seizures.[31] These similarities suggest that onset seizures after stroke and traumatic brain injury may have a common pathogenesis.[34 35] The risk of later seizures is, if anything, higher after stroke,[19] but such seizures are less likely to recur.[31]

Post stroke seizures

The risk of post stroke seizures was lower after cerebral infarction than after primary intracerebral haemorrhage or subarachnoid haemorrhage except among patients surviving total anterior circulation infarction, who had a 34% (12% to 57%) risk at 2 years. This estimated risk has broad confidence intervals because only 56 of these patients survived beyond the first 30 days, but it is significantly higher than after other subtypes of cerebral infarction. Post stroke seizures have previously been associated with severe paralytic stroke,[36] particularly when the cerebral cortex has been involved.[29] The increased incidence after total anterior circulation infarction may reflect the extensive damage frequently sustained to the frontal and temporal cortex, the most epileptogenic areas of the brain.[37]

Some patients in the Oxfordshire study developed post stroke seizures without any clinical or computed tomography evidence of cortical damage. Five patients developed post stroke seizures after lacunar infarction. One of these patients had a history of alcohol misuse and another had a dementing illness with evidence on postmortem examination of previous asymptomatic cerebral infarction. In the remaining three patients no other cause was found apart from the lacunar stroke. Other reports of seizures complicating basal ganglionic haemorrhage[38 39] and lacunar infarction[40] suggest that the association between post stroke seizures and cortical damage may not to be as exclusive as previously thought.[36]

The relative and cumulative risks of seizures after cerebral infarction were greater in the Oxfordshire community stroke project than in the one comparable study from Rochester,[19] but both these studies showed a significant excess risk in the first year after stroke and a similar reduction in relative risk with increasing age. The differences may be due to chance alone (the

Table 4 Post stroke seizures observed in the Oxfordshire community stroke project cohort over the first 2 years compared with the number expected to occur in the general population[10]

Age (years)	All strokes		Cerebral infarction	
	No observed	Observed/expected (95% CI)	No observed	Observed/expected (95% CI)
First year after stroke				
<65 (n=163)	9	104.2 (47.7 to 197.9)	5	75.9 (24.7 to 177.2)
65-74 (n=195)	5	22.6 (7.3 to 52.6)	5	27.3 (8.9 to 63.8)
>74 (n=317)	14	28.7 (15.7 to 48.2)	9	22.3 (10.2 to 42.4)
Total (n=675)	28	35.2 (23.4 to 50.9)	19	29.2 (17.6 to 45.5)
Second year after stroke				
<65 (n=129)	1	14.8 (0.4 to 82.6)	1	17.2 (0.4 to 95.8)
65-74 (n=154)	3	17.1 (3.5 to 50.1)	3	18.5 (3.8 to 54.0)
>74 (n=184)	6	21.2 (7.8 to 46.2)	6	23.2 (8.5 to 50.5)
Total (n=467)	10	19.0 (9.1 to 35.0)	10	21.0 (10.0 to 38.4)

Rochester results are all within the 95% confidence intervals of the estimates from the Oxfordshire study), but it is possible that the Oxfordshire study detected seizures that did not come to medical attention and so would not be included in the Rochester records.

Implications

Although the Oxfordshire study recorded an 11.5% risk of having a post stroke seizure by 5 years, a much higher risk than in the general population, almost half of these patients had only a single seizure, and of the 25 who had recurrent seizures only eight were having them frequently. It is unusual for epilepsy to be a major problem among stroke survivors,[29 32] and the risk of seizures in this study was significant only after a haemorrhagic or severe ischaemic stroke. Stroke survivors who were functionally independent at 1 or 6 months after the stroke had a very low risk of future seizures. The results suggest a cautious approach to instituting anticonvulsant treatment and support the current British licensing regulations which allow stroke patients who are functionally competent to return to driving after 30 days.

Appendix

A *single seizure* includes a single episode of status epilepticus or multiple seizures with less than 2 weeks between events. Seizures which were "provoked" by a stroke recurrence, occurring at the onset of a new cerebrovascular event, were included as post stroke seizures but were not included in the definition of recurrent seizures.

Recurrent seizures—two or more unprovoked seizures with at least two weeks between events.[29]

Prestroke seizure—single or recurrent seizures occurring before the day of the first stroke.

Onset seizures—seizures occurring within 24 hours of stroke onset or, in two cases, at three and four days during the evolution of a progressive stroke while it was still getting worse.

Post stroke seizures—seizures occuring more than 24 hours after stroke onset or after a stable deficit had been established.

We gratefully acknowledge support from the Medical Research Council (UK) and the Stroke Association. We also thank Lesley Jones, computer programmer, for her work in data management and statistical analysis, and the study nurses Sue Price, Liz Mogridge, and Claire Clifford. The project would not have been possible without the cooperation of the following general practices (liaison partners): Beaumont Street, Oxford (Dr A MacPherson); East Oxford Health Centre (Dr D Leggate); Thame (Dr A Marcus); Berinsfield (Dr M Agass); Stert Street, Abingdon (Dr N Crossley); Marcham Road, Abingdon (Dr R Pinches); Malthouse, Abingdon (Dr D Otterburn); Kidlington (Dr S Street); Wantage (Dr V Drury); Deddington (Dr H O'Donell). We also thank Mr Jim Slattery for statistical advice.

Funding: MRC and the Stroke Association.

Conflict of interest: None.

1 Roberts R, Shorvon S, Cox T, Gilliatt R. Clinically unsuspected cerebral infarction revealed by CT scanning in late onset epilepsy. *Epilepsia* 1988;29:190-4.

2 Roberts M, Godfrey J, Caird F. Epileptic seizures in the elderly: aetiology and type of seizure. *Age Ageing* 1982;11:24-8.

3 Bamford J, Sandercock P, Warlow C, Gray M. Why are patients with acute stroke admitted to hospital. *BMJ* 1986;292:1369-72.

4 Bamford J, Sandercock P, Dennis M, Warlow C, Jones L, McPherson K, et al. A prospective study of acute cerebrovascular disease in the community: the Oxfordshire community stroke project 1981-1986. *J Neurol Neurosurg Psychiatry* 1988;51:1373-80.

5 Bamford J, Sandercock P, Dennis M, Burn J, Warlow C. A prospective study of acute cerebrovascular disease in the community: the Oxfordshire community stroke project 1981-1986. Part 2. Incidence, case fatality rates and overall outcome at one year of cerebral infarction, primary intracerebral haemorrhage and subarachnoid haemorrhage. *J Neurol Neurosurg Psychiatry* 1990;53:16-22.

6 Bamford J, Sandercock P, Dennis M, Burn J, Warlow C. Classification and natural history of clinically identifiable subtypes of cerebral infarction. *Lancet* 1991;337:1521-6.

7 Bamford J, Warlow C. Evolution and testing of the lacunar hypothesis. *Stroke* 1988;19:1074-82.

8 Baquis GD, Pessin MS, Scott RM. Limb shaking—a carotid TIA. *Stroke* 1985;16:444-8.

9 Ropper AH. "Convulsions" in basilar artery occlusion. *Neurology* 1988;38:1500-1.

10 Bamford JM, Sandercock PAG, Warlow CP, Slattery J. Interobserver agreement for the assessment of handicap in stroke patients. *Stroke* 1989;20:828.

11 Annegers JF, Grabow JD, Groover RV, Laws ER, Elveback LR, Kurland LT. Seizures after head trauma: a population study. *Neurology* 1980;30:683-9.

12 Tallis R, Hall G, Craig I, Dean A. How common are epileptic seizures in old age? *Age Ageing* 1991;20:442-8.

13 Hall GC, Luscombe DK, Walker SR. Post-marketing surveillance using a computerised general practice database. *Pharm Med* 1988; 2:345-51.

14 Peto R, Pike MC, Armitage P, Breslow NE, Cox DR, Howard SV, et al. Design and analysis of randomised clinical trials requiring prolonged observation of each patient. 2. Analysis and examples. *Br J Cancer* 1977;35:1-39.

15 Gardner MJ, Altman DG, eds. *Statistics with confidence.* London: BMJ, 1989.

16 Moskowitz E, Lightbody FEH, Freitag NS. Long term follow up of the poststroke patient. *Arch Phys Med Rehabil* 1972;53:167-72.

17 Hauser WA, Ramirez-Lassepas H, Rosenstein R. Risk for seizures and epilepsy following cerebrovascular insults [abstract]. *Epilepsia* 1984;25:666.

18 Viitanen M, Erikson S, Asplund K. Risk of recurrent stroke, myocardial infarction and epilepsy during long term follow up after stroke. *Eur Neurol* 1988;28:227-31.

19 So E, Annegers J, Hauser W, O'Brien P, Whisnant M. Population-based study of seizure disorders after cerebral infarction. *Neurology* 1996;46:350-5.

20 Bamford J, Sandercock P, Warlow C, Gray M. Why are patients with acute stroke admitted to hospital? *BMJ* 1986;292:1369-72.

21 Barolin GS, Scherzer E, Schnaberth G. Epileptische Manifestationen als Vorboten von Schlaganfällen. "Vaskuläre Präkursiv Epilepsie." *Fortschr Neurol Psychiatr* 1971;39:199-216.

22 Goodridge DMG, Shorvon SD. Epileptic seizures in a population of 6000. 1. Demography, diagnosis, and classification and role of the hospital services. *BMJ* 1983;287:641-4.

23 Shinton RA, Gill JS, Zezulka AV, Beevers DG. The frequency of epilepsy preceding stroke. *Lancet* 1987;1:11-3.

24 Starkey IR, Warlow CP. Epilepsy preceding stroke [letter]. *Lancet* 1987;1:742-3.

25 Kase CS, Wolf PA, Chodosh EH, Zacker HB, Kelly-Hayes M, Kannel WB, et al. Prevalence of silent stroke in patients with initial stroke: the Framingham study. *Stroke* 1989;20:850-2.

26 Shinton RA, Gill JS, Melnick SC, Gupta AK, Beevers DG. The frequency, characteristics and prognosis of epileptic seizures at the onset of stroke. *J Neurol Neurosurg Psychiatry* 1988;51:273-6.

27 Davalos A, Cendra E, Genis D, Lopez-Pousa S. The frequency, characteristics and prognosis of epileptic seizures at the onset of stroke [letter]. *J Neurol Neurosurg Psychiatry* 1988;51:1464.

28 Aring CD, Merrit HH. Differential diagnosis between cerebral haemorrhage and cerebral thrombosis. *Arch Intern Med* 1935;56:435-56.

29 Kilpatrick CJ, Davis SM, Tress BM, Rossiter SC, Hopper JL, Vandendriesen ML. Epileptic seizures in acute stroke. *Arch Neurol* 1990;47:157-60.

30 Reith J, Jorgensen HS, Nakayama H, Raascha HO, Olsen TS. Early seizures do not worsen rehabilitation outcome. The Copenhagen stroke study [abstract]. *Eur J Neurol* 1996;3(suppl 2):93.

31 Jennet B. *Epilepsy after non-missile head injury.* London: Whitefriars Press, 1975.

32 Gupta SR, Naheedy MN, Elias D, Rubino FA. Postinfarction seizures: a clinical study. *Stroke* 1988;19:1477-81.

33 De Carolis P, D'Alessandro RD, Ferrara R, Andreoli A, Saquegna T, Lugaresi E. Late seizures in patients with internal carotid artery and middle cerebral artery occlusive disease following ischaemic events. *J Neurol Neurosurg Psychiatry* 1984;47:1345-7.

34 Dodge PR, Richardson EP, Victor M. Recurrent convulsive seizures as a sequel to cerebral infarction: a clinical and pathological study. *Brain* 1954;77:610-46.

35 Evans JH. The significance of early post-traumatic epilepsy. *Neurology* 1963;13:207-12.

36 Olsen TS, Hogenhaven H, Thage O. Epilepsy after stroke. *Neurology* 1987;37:1209-11.

37 French JD, Gernandt BE, Livingstone RB. Regional differences in seizure susceptibility in monkey cortex. *Arch Neurol Psychiatr* 1956;75:260-74.

38 Faught E, Peters D. Seizures in intracerebral haemorrhage [abstract]. *Epilepsia* 1984;25:666.

39 Sung C-Y, Chu N-S. Epileptic seizures in intracerebral haemorrhage. *J Neurol Neurosurg Psychiatry* 1989;52:1273-6.

40 Avrahami A, Drury VE, Rabey MJ, Cohn DF. Generalised epileptic seizures as the presenting symptom of lacunar infarction in the brain. *J Neurol* 1988;235:472-4.

(Accepted 8 July 1997)

Citation:

Are the results of this prognosis study valid?

Was a defined, representative sample of patients
assembled at a common (usually early) point in
the course of their disease?

Was patient follow-up sufficiently long and
complete?

Were objective outcome criteria applied in a
'blind' fashion?

If subgroups with different prognoses are identified,
was there adjustment for important prognostic
factors?

Was there validation in an independent group
('test-set') of patients?

Are the valid results of this prognosis study important?

How likely are the outcomes over time?

How precise are the prognostic estimates?

If you want to calculate a confidence interval around the measure of prognosis

(see Appendix 1 in *Evidence-based Medicine*)

Clinical Measure	Standard Error (SE)	Typical calculation of CI
Proportion (as in the rate of some prognostic event, etc.) where: the number of patients = n the proportion of these patients who experience the event = p	$\sqrt{\{p \times (1-p)/n\}}$ where p is proportion and n is number of patients	If p = 24/60 = 0.4 (or 40%) and n = 60 $SE = \sqrt{\{0.4 \times (1-0.4)/60\}}$ = 0.063 (or 6.3%) 95% CI is 40% +/– 1.96 x 6.3% or 27.6% to 52.4%
n from your evidence: _____ p from your evidence: _____	$\sqrt{\{p \times (1-p)/n\}}$ where p is proportion and n is number of patients	Your calculation: SE: _____ 95% CI: _____

Can you apply this valid, important evidence about prognosis in caring for your patient?

Were the study patients similar to your own?

Will this evidence make a clinically important impact on your conclusions about what to offer or tell your patient?

Additional notes

Citation: Burn J, Dennis M, Bamford J *et al.* (1997) Epileptic seizures after a first stroke: the Oxfordshire Community Stroke Project. *BMJ.* 315: 1582–7.

Are the results of this prognosis study valid?

Was a defined, representative sample of patients assembled at a common (usually early) point in the course of their disease?	**Yes. From a common starting point but we don't know how GPs decided which stroke patients to send to hospital.**
Was patient follow-up sufficiently long and complete?	**Yes. For a minimum of 2 years and up to 6.5 years.**
Were objective outcome criteria applied in a 'blind' fashion?	**Patients were asked at follow-up if they had a seizure and were then assessed by a study neurologist (not sure if neurologist was blinded).**
If subgroups with different prognoses are identified, was there adjustment for important prognostic factors?	**Looked at different stroke types and previous history of stroke.**
Was there validation in an independent group ('test-set') of patients?	**No.**

Are the valid results of this prognosis study important?

How likely are the outcomes over time?	**5.7% over one year.**
How precise are the prognostic estimates?	**95% confidence interval – 3.5% to 7.9%.**

If you want to calculate a confidence interval around the measure of prognosis

(see Appendix 1 in *Evidence-based Medicine*)

Clinical Measure	Standard Error (SE)	Typical calculation of CI
Proportion (as in the rate of some prognostic event, etc.) where: the number of patients = n the proportion of these patients who experience the event = p	$\sqrt{\{p \times (1-p)/n\}}$ where p is proportion and n is number of patients	If p = 24/60 = 0.4 (or 40%) and n = 60 $SE = \sqrt{\{0.4 \times (1-0.4)/60\}}$ = 0.063 (or 6.3%) 95% CI is 40% +/– 1.96 x 6.3% or 27.6% to 52.4%
n from your evidence: **675** p from your evidence: **0.**	$\sqrt{\{p \times (1-p)/n\}}$ where p is proportion and n is number of patients	Your calculation: SE: **0.009** 95% CI: **5.7% +/– 1.7% = 4% to 7.4%**

Can you apply this valid, important evidence about prognosis in caring for your patient?

Were the study patients similar to your own?	**Yes.**
Will this evidence make a clinically important impact on your conclusions about what to offer or tell your patient?	**Yes.**

Additional notes

STROKE – RISK OF SEIZURE

Appraised by Sharon Straus:
March 1998.
Expiry date: 2000.

Clinical Bottom Line

Stroke patients have a 5.7% risk of seizure at one year.

Citation

Burn J, Dennis M, Bamford J *et al.* (1997) Epileptic seizures after a first stroke: the Oxfordshire Community Stroke Project. *BMJ*. **315**: 1582–7.

Three-part Question

In a patient with stroke, what is the risk of seizure at one year?

Search Terms

'stroke' and 'seizure' in MEDLINE.

The Study

675 pts registered in a community-based stroke registry after their first stroke.

The Outcome: seizure.

Well-defined sample at uniform (early) stage of illness? – Yes; Follow-up long enough? – Yes; Follow-up complete? – Yes; Blind and objective outcome criteria? – No; Adjustment for other prognostic factors? – No; Validation in an independent 'test-set' of patients? – No.

The Evidence

Prognostic Factor	Outcome	Time	Measure	Confidence Interval
Cerebral infarction	Seizure	One year	4.2%	2.2 to 6.2%
Primary intracerebral haemorrhage	Seizure	One year	20%	1.5 to 38.3%
Subarachnoid haemorrhage	Seizure	One year	22%	2.6 to 41.8%
Any stroke	Seizure	One year	5.7%	3.5 to 7.9%

Comments

1. Unsure how physicians selected patients for registration.
2. Onset seizures (those occurring within 24 hours of onset of stroke) associated with increased risk of seizure – OR 7.52 (2.46 to 22.98).
3. Probability of post-stroke seizure higher among patients >84 (but numbers small).

4

Harm and searching the primary literature

PART A   Critical appraisal of a clinical article about harm

You see a 73-year old man in your general medicine clinic who has a history of hypertension for which he has been taking nifedipine XL 30 mg PO per day for 5 years. In his retirement he has learned how to use the Internet, and he brings you a print-out of some newspaper headlines that he unearthed while surfing the net:

'Hypertension Med Kills'
LA Times

'Drug for blood pressure linked to heart attacks: researchers fear 6 million are imperilled'
Washington Post

He is very worried and wants to know if he should stop taking nifedipine. Together, you form the clinical question: 'In patients taking calcium antagonists for hypertension, do these calcium antagonists cause cancer?' You track down the *Lancet* article referred to in the scary newspaper article (*Lancet* (1996) **348:** 493–7).

Read this article and decide:
1   Are the results of this harm study valid?
2   Are the results of this harm study important?
3   Should these valid, important results of this study about a potentially harmful treatment change the treatment of your patient?

If you want to read some strategies for answering these sorts of questions, see pp 105–10, 147–9 and 179–81 in *Evidence-based Medicine*

PART B   Searching for evidence in the primary literature

Colleagues from the library will whet your appetite for learning how to search for evidence in the clinical literature (or hone the searching skills you have already developed), so bring along the clinical questions you generated in Session 2 (or any that you have generated in the meantime). Efficient EBM searching strategies (that trade off the sensitivity and specificity of your searches) are included.

BEST SINGLE TERMS AND COMBINATIONS FOR HIGH SENSITIVITY MEDLINE SEARCHES ON THE BEST STUDIES OF TREATMENT, DIAGNOSIS, PROGNOSIS, OR CAUSE.

Search strategy	Sensitivity[1]	Specificity	Precision
For studies of treatment:			
Clinical trial (pt)	0.93	0.92	0.49
Randomised controlled trial (pt) or Drug therapy (sh) or Therapeutic use (sh) or Random: (tw)	0.99	0.74	0.22
For studies of prognosis:			
Exp cohort Studies	0.60	0.80	0.11
Incidence or Exp mortality or Follow up studies or Mortality: (sh) or Prognosis: (tw) or Predict: (tw) or Course (tw)	0.92	0.73	0.11
For studies of aetiology or cause:			
Risk (tw)	0.67	0.79	0.15
Exp cohort studies or Exp risk or Odds and ratio: (tw) or Relative and risk: (tw) or Case and control: (tw)	0.82	0.70	0.14
For studies of diagnosis:			
Diagnosis (pe)	0.80	0.77	0.09
Exp Sensitivity and specificity or Diagnosis: (pe) or Diagnostic use or Sensitivity: (tw) or Specificity: (tw)	0.92	0.73	0.09

[1]**Sensitivity**, as defined in the study on which the table is based, is the proportion of studies in MEDLINE meeting criteria for scientific soundness and clinical relevance that are detected. **Specificity** is the proportion of less sound/relevant studies that are excluded by the search strategy. **Precision** is the proportion of all citations retrieved that are both sound and relevant. (Source: *Evidence-based Medicine*; also see the Web pages.)

Articles

Calcium-channel blockade and incidence of cancer in aged populations

Marco Pahor, Jack M Guralnik, Luigi Ferrucci, Maria-Chiara Corti, Marcel E Salive, James R Cerhan,
Robert B Wallace, Richard J Havlik

Summary

Background Calcium-channel blockers can alter apoptosis, a mechanism for destruction of cancer cells. We examined whether the long-term use of calcium-channel blockers is associated with an increased risk of cancer.

Methods Between 1988 and 1992 we carried out a prospective cohort study of 5052 people aged 71 years or more and who lived in three regions of Massachusetts, Iowa, and Connecticut USA. Those taking calcium-channel blockers (n=451) were compared with all other participants (n=4601). The incidence of cancer was assessed by survey of hospital discharge diagnoses and causes of death. These outcomes were validated by the cancer registry in the one region where it was available. Demographic variables, disability, cigarette smoking, alcohol consumption, blood pressure, body-mass index, use of other drugs, hospital admissions for other causes, and comorbidity were all assessed as possible confounding factors.

Findings The hazard ratio for cancer associated with calcium-channel blockers (1549 person-years, 47 events) compared with those not taking calcium-channel blockers (17 225 person-years, 373 events) was 1·72 (95% CI 1·27–2·34, p=0·0005), after adjustment for confounding factors. A significant dose-response gradient was found. Hazard ratios associated with verapamil, diltiazem, and nifedipine did not differ significantly from each other. The results remained unchanged in community-specific analyses. The association between calcium-channel blockers and cancer was found with most of the common cancers.

Interpretation Calcium-channel blockers were associated with a general increased risk of cancer in the study populations, which suggested a common mechanism. These observational findings should be confirmed by other studies.

Lancet 1996; **348**: 493–97

See Editorial page 487

See Commentary pages 488 and 489

Introduction

Calcium-channel blockers are prescribed primarily for

Department of Internal Medicine and Geriatrics, Catholic University, Rome, Italy (M Pahor MD); **Epidemiology, Demography, and Biometry Program, National Institute on Aging, Bethesda, MD, USA** (J M Guralnik MD, M-C Corti MD, M E Salive MD, R J Havlik MD); **Geriatric Department, I Fraticini, Istituto Nazionale Ricerca e Cura Per Gli Anziani (INRCA), Florence, Italy** (L Ferrucci MD); **and Department of Preventive Medicine and Environmental Health, University of Iowa, IA, USA** (J R Cerhan MD, R B Wallace MD)

Correspondence to: Dr Marco Pahor, Department of Preventive Medicine, University of Tennessee, Memphis, 66 N Pauline, Suite 232, Memphis, TN 38105, USA

treatment of hypertension and coronary heart disease but lately their long-term safety has been questioned.[1-4] Excess all-cause mortality has been associated with the use of short-acting nifedipine.[1,2] Calcium-channel blockers are potent drugs that affect various organ systems. Calcium-channel blockers are used to treat oesophageal diseases,[5] and cause constipation,[6] increase risk of haemorrhage,[7,8] and can impair differentiation during embryogenesis.[9] Furthermore, cases of lupus after use of diltiazem have been reported.[10]

We have hypothesised that calcium-channel blockers increase the risk of cancer by interfering with physiological mechanisms that regulate cancer cell growth.[4,11] Evidence is emerging that calcium-channel blockers can block apoptosis,[12-14] an efficient mechanism for limiting cancer growth.[15-18] Calcium-channel blockers might affect cancer risk generally or be limited to specific sites where calcium mechanisms predominate. For example, colon cancer has been related to reduced calcium ingestion.[19]

In this prospective study, the initial analyses done in individuals receiving treatment for hypertension[11] have been extended to the general older population. The aim was to assess whether individuals taking calcium-channel blockers, for any indication were at higher risk of developing cancer than those not taking those drugs. The study focused on specific cancers, additional potential confounding factors, and the effects of dose.

Methods

The study was based on the Established Populations for Epidemiologic Studies of the Elderly (EPESE)—a collaborative, prospective cohort study of older persons supported by the US National Institute on Aging.[20] The participants surveyed were from three regions. Between 1982 and 1983, a regional survey was carried out on all persons aged 65 years or older living in East Boston, Massachusetts, and in the counties of Iowa and Washington in the state of Iowa. During the same period of time another survey was done in New Haven, Connecticut, where a random sample stratified by housing type and sex was taken.

Over 80% of the eligible population was interviewed. At the initial EPESE interview, and after 3 and 6 years of follow-up, trained interviewers administered a 90-min questionnaire that covered a wide range of psychosocial and health-related issues. Telephone follow-up interviews were done 1, 2, 4, and 5 years after the initial interview. Cancer events were assessed for the time between the sixth EPESE annual follow-up in 1988 and the end of 1992.

Information on date of hospital admission and up to five discharge diagnoses for each person in the survey was gathered from the Health Care Financing Administration Medicare Provider Analysis and Review (MEDPAR) files. The match of EPESE participants with MEDPAR files was complete from Jan 1, 1985, until Dec 31, 1992.

Vital status on Dec 31, 1992, was assessed at the seventh follow-up (Iowa and Connecticut) by contact with relatives, examination of obituaries in local newspapers, and linkage with the National Death Index.[21] One nosologist studied death certificates and then used ICD-9 codes to record the underlying, immediate, and contributing causes of death. Hospital discharge diagnoses or causes of death with ICD-9 codes 140–208 recorded at any time in the MEDPAR files were defined as cancer events. Specific codes were used to identify site of cancer.

In previous studies, hospital chart reviews provided validation of cancer as a hospital discharge diagnosis.[22] In this study, in the individuals from the Iowa regions cancer outcomes were validated by matching of the EPESE participants with the State Health Registry of Iowa's cancer registry, which is part of the National Cancer Institute's Surveillance, Epidemiology, and End Results (SEER) program.[23] The kappa statistic[24] for the agreement of the MEDPAR files and death certificates with the SEER registry in ascertaining prevalent (before baseline), incident, and any prevalent or incident cancer cases was 0·77, 0·83, and 0·86, respectively.

During the section of the baseline interview on the use of medications, participants were asked to show all containers for all prescription and non-prescription drugs taken over the past 2 weeks. The interviewer transcribed the drug product name from the container label. If the label was not seen, the interviewer asked the participant the name of the drug. These ascertainment methods are similar to those of other studies and have proven valid and reliable.[25,26] Participants taking calcium-channel blockers were compared with participants who were not. In addition, separate analyses were done for verapamil, nifedipine, and diltiazem.

For participants living in Massachussetts and Iowa the daily dose of calcium-channel blocker was calculated; the strength of the drug product was multiplied by the number of times the medication was taken per day. In Connecticut the dose could not be calculated. The median dose was established for verapamil, nifedipine, and diltiazem separately (240, 30, and 180 mg/day, respectively), then the calcium-channel blocker dose was ranked as low (below median), median, or high (over median).

The following factors potentially associated with cancer were assessed at the baseline interview: age; sex; ethnic origin; coronary heart disease (use of nitrates, self-report of heart attack, any hospital discharge diagnosis coded 410–414 in the preceding 3 years, or a positive Rose questionnaire for angina assessed at any interview giving in person[27]); heart failure (use of both digoxin and a diuretic, or any hospital discharge diagnosis coded 428 in the preceding 3 years); hypertension (systolic blood pressure ≥140 mm Hg or diastolic ≥90 mm Hg measured at any visit, self-report of a medical diagnosis of hypertension, or any hospital discharge diagnosis coded 401 in the preceding 3 years); stroke (self-report of stroke, or any hospital discharge diagnosis coded 430–434 in the preceding 3 years); diabetes (use of antidiabetic drugs, self-report of diabetes, or any hospital discharge diagnosis coded 250 in the preceding 3 years); use of β-blockers, angiotensin-converting enzyme (ACE) inhibitors, diuretics, digoxin, nitrates, non-steroidal anti-inflammatory drugs, aspirin, corticosteroids, oestrogens, or coumarin; current smoking status (non-smoker or smoking 1–19 or ≥20 cigarettes per day); alcohol intake (≥28·35 g/day, assessed by self-reported frequency and number of consumed drinks of beer, wine, and spirits); and physical disability (limitation in one or more of the following: walking half a mile, climbing a flight of stairs, doing heavy housework, walking across a room, bathing, dressing, eating, or transferring from bed to chair).[28,29] Trained interviewers measured blood pressure two or three times according to the Hypertension Detection and Follow-up Program protocol.[30] The mean of the last two measurements was calculated. Body-mass index was calculated from reported weight and height. The number of hospital admissions before the qualifying event or before the end of follow-up was assessed.

Of the original population of more than 10 000 interviewed in 1982, 6566 participants were still alive and were interviewed in 1988, the baseline period for this study. We excluded 298 participants who could not be matched with MEDPAR files, and 1216 participants who reported a cancer at any of the interviews, who had a hospital discharge diagnosis of cancer in the 3 years

Characteristic	Not taking calcium-channel blockers (n=4601)	Taking calcium-channel blockers (n=451)	p*
Demographic			
Mean (SE) age	79·3 (0·1)	79·0 (0·3)	p>0·1
Women	64·5%	64·1%	p>0·1
Ethic origin			
White	94·2%	93·6%	
Black	5·1%	6·4%	p>0·1
Other	0·7%	0	
Comorbid conditions			
Coronary heart disease	21·9%	71·2%	p<0·0001
Heart failure	9·7%	29·3%	p<0·0001
Hypertension	81·7%	90·0%	p<0·0001
Stroke	9·2%	12·6%	p=0·016
Diabetes	15·7%	26·2%	p<0·0001
Medications			
β-blockers	11·6%	23·3%	p<0·0001
ACE inhibitors	4·4%	8·6%	p<0·0001
Diuretics	33·5%	50·6%	p<0·0001
Digoxin	11·6%	25·1%	p<0·0001
Nitrates	6·2%	38·8%	p<0·0001
NSAIDs	12·5%	14·6%	p>0·1
Aspirin	29·7%	37·3%	p<0·001
Oestrogens	0·8%	0·2%	p>0·1
Corticosteroids	3·2%	3·8%	p>0·1
Coumarin	2·6%	6·0%	p<0·0001
Mean (SE) blood pressure (mm Hg)			
Systolic	136 (0·4)	138 (1·3)	p>0·1
Diastolic	73 (0·2)	72 (0·6)	p=0·033
Mean (SE) body-mass index (kg/m²)	24·4 (0·1)	24·8 (0·3)	p>0·1
Smoking status			
Current non-smoker	90·1%	91·8%	p>0·1
1–19 cigarettes per day	4·9%	5·3%	
≥20 cigarettes per day	3·8%	2·7%	
Alcohol intake			
≥28·35 g per day	5·0%	4·4%	p>0·1
Health indicators			
Physical disability	45·4%	62·7%	p<0·0001
Mean (SE) number of hospital admissions	1·2 (0)	2·2 (0·1)	p<0·0001

Percentages may not total 100% because of missing data. *χ² test for categorical variables, ANOVA or Mann-Whitney tests for comparison of means. ACE=angiotensin converting enzyme. NSAIDs=non-steroidal anti-inflammatory drugs.

Table 1: **Population baseline characteristics according to use of calcium-channel blockers**

before the study baseline, or who were taking anticancer drugs such as tamoxifen. The remaining population at risk was 5052 participants (1741 from East Boston, 2020 from Iowa, and 1291 from New Haven).

The first cancer event that occurred during follow-up was used as a primary endpoint. Participants with no events, by the time of the final follow-up in 1992 were censored on Dec 31, 1992, or at the time of death, whichever occurred first. The Kaplan-Meier method was used to plot survival free of cancer. Cox proportional hazards regression models were used to estimate the hazard ratio and 95% CI for the association of variables of interest with cancer. The assumption of proportionality of hazard was assessed with log minus log plots and by tests of the interaction of exposure with time. In multivariate models, additional indicator variables were created to adjust for the effects of missing data for cigarette smoking, alcohol intake, and disability (1·1%, 0·8%, and 6·8% with missing data, respectively). In analyses summarising results for all three regions, the regression models were stratified by region.

Results

Compared with participants who were not taking calcium-channel blockers those taking these drugs were significantly more likely to have cardiovascular diseases and diabetes, to use cardiovascular drugs, to be disabled, to have a lower diastolic blood pressure, and to be

	Number of events	Person-years	Rate per 1000 person-years	Unadjusted model		Adjusted model*	
				Hazard ratio (95% CI)	p	Hazard ratio (95% CI)	p
All calcium-channel blockers							
Non-users (n=4601)	373	17 225	21·7	1	..	1	..
Users (n=451)	47	1549	30·3	1·42 (1·05–1·92)	0·032	1·72 (1·27–2·34)	0·0005
Individual calcium-channel blockers							
Verapamil (n=118)	18	420	42·9	2·03 (1·26–3·25)	0·0035	2·49 (1·54–4·01)	0·0002
Nifedipine (n=146)	16	480	33·3	1·56 (0·94–2·51)	0·083	1·74 (1·05–2·88)	0·031
Diltiazem (n=184)	13	641	20·3	0·94 (0·54–1·63)	>0·1	1·22 (0·70–2·12)	>0·1

*Adjusted for age, sex, ethnic origin, heart failure, number of hospital admissions, cigarette smoking, and alcohol intake. Three participants were excluded from the analyses of individual calcium-channel blockers because they were taking two calcium-channel blockers.

Table 2: **Use of calcium-channel blockers and their relation to cancer**

admitted to hospital (table 1). Age, sex, ethnic origin, cigarette smoking, alcohol intake, systolic blood pressure, body-mass index, and use of non-cardiovascular drugs did not differ significantly between the two groups.

During 18 774 person-years of follow-up (mean follow-up time 3·7 years), 420 participants had a cancer event (140 in East Boston, 185 in Iowa, and 95 in New Haven; overall rate 22·4 per 1000 person-years; table 2). The most frequent cancers were those of the colon, prostate, lung, lymphatic and haemopoietic organs, urinary tract, and breast (table 3). 169 people died from cancer (9·0 per 1000 person-years).

Users of calcium-channel blockers had significantly higher crude rates of cancer than non-users (table 2, figure 1). Patients taking verapamil had the highest rate of cancer followed by patients taking nifedipine and diltiazem.

To assess independent risk factors for cancer that might have confounded the association of calcium-channel blockers with cancer, separate proportional hazard regression models (adjusted for age and sex) were calculated for groups of variables, including demographic characteristics, chronic diseases, medications, and general health indicators (cigarette smoking, alcohol intake, physical disability, blood pressure, body-mass index, and number of hospital admissions). In the initial models there were significant associations between age, being male, being black, cigarette smoking, and alcohol consumption and increased risk of cancer. An inverse relation with cancer was found for heart failure and number of hospital admissions (p<0·1). In a summary multivariate model adjusted for these potential confounding factors, calcium-channel blocker users had a

significantly increased risk of cancer compared with all other participants (hazard ratio=1·72, p=0·0005, table 2). The association was significant for verapamil and nifedipine, but not for diltiazem. However, the difference in hazard ratio among specific calcium-channel blockers was not significant. In the fully adjusted models the hazard ratios were greater than those calculated without adjustment. In separate models adjusted for confounding factors and either systolic and diastolic blood pressure or any past diagnosis of hypertension, the hazard ratio of cancer associated with calcium-channel blockers was 1·67 (1·21–2·29), and 1·71 (1·25–2·32), respectively. The hazard ratio associated with use of β-blockers, ACE inhibitors, diuretics, digoxin, nitrates, non-steroidal anti-inflammatory drugs, aspirin, corticosteroids, or coumarin was not significant and was close to 1 (not shown).

In community-specific multivariate analyses, the hazard ratio of cancer for calcium-channel blocker users was 1·55 (0·89–2·71), 1·82 (1·12–2·98), and 1·84 (1·04–3·26), compared with all other participants, in East Boston, Iowa, and New Haven, respectively. Daily dose of calcium-channel blocker was assessed in East Boston and Iowa and increasing dose was associated with a significant gradient of increased hazard ratio of cancer when compared with those who did not use calcium-channel blockers (figure 2).

Separate multivariate models stratified according to potential risk factors of cancer were calculated. The hazard ratio of cancer for calcium-channel blockers was 1·77 (1·20–2·63) in participants aged 71–79 years (n=2982) and 1·55 (0·93–2·59) in those aged 80 years and older (n=2070); 1·64 (1·09–2·46) in men (n=1796) and 1·81 (1·13–2·90) in women (n=3256); 1·60 (1·15–2·22) in white people (n=4757) and 3·42 (1·25–9·39) in black people (n=264); 1·78 (1·29–2·47) in those not currently cigarette smokers (n=4559) and 1·44 (0·55–3·73) in current cigarette smokers (n=439); 1·76 (1·27–2·42) in those drinking <28·35 g of alcohol per day (n=4762) and 1·26 (0·42–3·73) in those drinking ≥28·35 g of alcohol per day (n=252); 1·71 (1·23–2·37) in those with any lifetime diagnosis of hypertension (n=4163) and 1·99 (0·78–5·07) in those with no hypertension (n=889); 1·80 (1·17–2·76) in those with diastolic and systolic blood pressure below 90 mm Hg and below 140 mm Hg, respectively (n=2313); and 1·57 (0·97–2·54) in those with elevated (≥90/140 mm Hg) blood pressure (n=1969).

In multivariate models stratified by number of hospital admissions, and in analyses that excluded cancer events in which a circulatory disease (ICD 9 codes 390–459) was the principal discharge diagnosis, the results for calcium-channel blockers were unchanged (summary hazard ratio for the stratified models 1·70 [1·25–2·31], and 1·62, [1·18–2·24], respectively). When individual cancer sites were analysed separately, calcium-channel blocker use

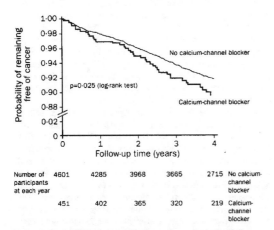

Figure 1: **Probability of remaining free of cancer during follow-up according to use of calcium-channel blockers**

Type of cancer (ICD-9 code)	Number of events	Hazard ratio (95% CI)
Stomach (151)	13	3·64 (0·96–13·76)
Colon (153)	65	1·98 (0·90–4·38)
Rectum (154)	23	1·32 (0·31–5·74)
Liver, gallbladder, pancreas (155–157)	24	1·15 (0·26–4·96)
Lung (162)	56	0·21 (0·03–1·52)
Skin (172–173)	14	1·11 (0·14–8·62)
Breast (174)	31	1·65 (0·49–5·55)*
Uterus, adnexa (182–183)	23	3·69 (1·22–11·14)*
Prostate (185)	58	1·99 (0·93–4·27)
Bladder, ureter, kidney (188–189)	38	1·57 (0·55–4·47)
Lymphatic, haemopoietic (200–208)	46	2·57 (1·13–5·83)

Regression models stratified by community and adjusted for age, sex, ethnic origin, heart failure, number of hospital admissions, cigarette smoking, and alcohol intake.
*Adjusted for oestrogen use.

Table 3: **Relation of use of calcium-channel blockers with specific types of cancer**

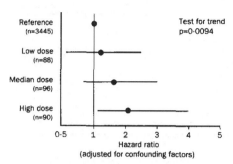

Figure 2: **Hazard ratio and 95% CI of incident cancer according to daily dose of calcium-channel blocker compared with no calcium-channel blocker use**
Estimates are adjusted for age, sex, ethnic origin, heart failure, number of hospital admissions, smoking, and alcohol intake. Median daily dose for verapamil, nifedipine, and diltiazem 240, 30, and 180 mg.

was associated with a significantly increased hazard ratio for cancers of the uterus and adnexa uteri, and lymphatic and haemopoietic organs (table 3). The hazard ratio was increased, but did not reach significance for stomach, colon, rectum, breast, prostate, and urinary tract cancers. For liver, gallbladder and pancreas, and skin cancers, the hazard ratio was increased, but close to 1. A non-significant inverse relation was found for lung cancer (table 3).

Separate analyses used the Iowa SEER cancer registry data rather than the MEDPAR files or death certificates to define the population that was free of cancer at baseline and incident cases of cancer. In these analyses, the incidence rate of cancer was 12·1 per 1000 person-years among participants not taking calcium-channel blockers (120 events, 1829 participants) and 30·4 per 1000 person-years among those taking calcium-channel blockers (16 events, 106 participants, p<0·001). After adjustment for confounding factors, the hazard ratio of cancer associated with calcium-channel blocker use was 3·09 (1·80–5·31), p<0·0001.

Discussion

We found that after adjustment for confounding factors, older people taking calcium-channel blockers for any indication had a significant 70% excess hazard ratio of developing cancer during 3·7 years (mean) of follow-up compared with those not taking these drugs. This association was consistent in all three regions in this study, and for most types of cancer. The dose-response gradient was significant. The excess risk of cancer associated with use of calcium-channel blockers was even more evident when the SEER cancer registry information was used to define the events. No association with cancer was found for other cardiovascular medications.

If calcium-channel blockers truly promote cancer, what are the potential mechanisms? Apoptosis, or programmed cell death, is an efficient physiological mechanism for elimination of cells with genetic lesions, and, therefore, for preventing cancer.[15] Calcium-channel blockers inhibit apoptosis in various experimental models by interfering with calcium-triggered signals.[12,14,18] At therapeutic concentrations, verapamil and nifedipine suppress gene activity associated with involution by apoptosis of prostate and breast after the removal of physiological hormone stimulation.[12,31] Such mechanisms may also prevent apoptosis of neoplastic cells, thereby promoting cancer growth.[11] Inhibition of calcium-mediated cell differentiation may also play a part.[18]

The consistent association of calcium-channel blockers with increase in most types of cancer found in this study suggests that calcium-channel blockers might promote cancer through a common underlying biological process, such as interference with apoptosis or cell differentiation. Calcium-channel blockers may act as cancer promoters but standard carcinogenicity bioassays, which are designed to identify chemical mutagens, may fail to recognise such promoters. Further research is needed to assess whether the inverse relation of calcium-channel blockers with lung cancer was produced by chance alone or by other specific mechanisms.

Calcium-channel blocker use was ascertained at baseline and the latent period required for producing a clinically relevant cancer could not be calculated. Interestingly the Kaplan-Meier curves start diverging at about 2 years after the start of the study. The latent period for the underlying mechanism by which calcium-channel blockers might promote cancer may be less than that needed for chemical mutagens.

Calcium-channel blockers can potentiate anticancer drugs and facilitate apoptosis. However, such effects were observed in animal and in-vitro models at toxic concentrations not tolerated in man, and were accompanied by a paradoxical increase in intracellular calcium.[32]

We have identified six potential limitations of the study. First, although several confounding factors were examined, observational data such as these cannot conclusively establish causal links. Whether calcium-channel blockers truly promote cancer needs to be confirmed in long-term clinical trials. Physical disabilities and the consequent incapacity of a number of participants in this study would probably preclude their attendance for follow-up visits. Thus, these individuals would probably be excluded from clinical trials.

Second, users of calcium-channel blockers had higher rates than the non-users of hospital admission for cardiovascular disease; this difference could have led to a bias in cancer detection. However, the significant calcium-channel blocker cancer association did not change after adjustment or stratification on number of hospital admissions, and after exclusion of cancer hospital admissions in which a circulatory disease was the principal diagnosis. Use of other antihypertensive agents, nitrates, digoxin, corticosteroids, and anticoagulants, which are used for treating diseases requiring frequent medical surveillance, was not associated with cancer.

Patients with heart failure, who are frequently admitted to hospital, tended to have a lower hazard ratio of cancer. Patients who are elderly and have an important cardiovascular condition might not undergo cancer screening as often as those who are healthy.

A third possible limitation was that exposure and outcome may have been misclassified. Drug use was assessed only at baseline and some participants may have stopped taking calcium-channel blockers during follow-up. Furthermore, cancers that did not lead to hospital admission or death were not ascertained, and the diagnoses in the MEDPAR files and death certificates may not be accurate. However, such potential misclassifications would probably dilute any associations found and introduce a conservative bias, leading to an underestimation of the association of calcium-channel blocker use with cancer.

Fourth, our findings in older people who have higher rates of cancer may not be applicable to younger individuals. Fifth, mainly short-acting calcium-channel blockers were used in this study. Theoretically, with new calcium-channel blockers and the slow-release formulations the plasma concentrations may remain below a harmful threshold. Finally, hypertension has been associated with an increased risk of cancer mortality in middle-aged people.[33,34] However, in this study blood pressure was not related to cancer and did not confound the calcium-channel blocker-cancer association.

Evaluation of long-term safety and efficacy of medications such as calcium-channel blockers, which exert multiple and incompletely identified actions, needs to focus on assessment of major outcomes and survival.[1-3,8,35,36] A judgment about the clinical implications of our findings is currently premature. The evidence provided by this single study is not sufficient to recommend withdrawal of treatment from current users. However, these observational data should stimulate further experimental, epidemiological, and clinical research to assess all the cardiovascular and non-cardiovascular effects of calcium-channel blockers.

This study was supported by contracts N01-AG-0-2105, N01-AG-0-2106, and N01-AG-0-2107 from the National Institute on Aging, Bethesda, MD, USA. MP was supported by a grant from Ministero per l'Università e Ricerca Scientifica e Tecnologica, 60% N7020532, and from Consiglio Nazionale delle Ricerche, Italy, N95000959PF40.

References

1 Pahor M, Guralnik JM, Corti C, Foley DJ, Carbonin PU, Havlik RJ. Long-term survival and use of antihypertensive medications in older persons. *J Am Geriatr Soc* 1995; 43: 1191–97.

2 Furberg CD, Psaty BM, Meyer JV. Nifedipine. Dose-related increase in mortality in patients with coronary heart disease. *Circulation* 1995; 92: 1326–31.

3 Psaty BM, Heckbert SR, Koepsell TD, et al. The risk of myocardial infarction associated with antihypertensive drug therapies. *JAMA* 1995; 274: 620–25.

4 Furberg CD, Pahor M, Psaty BM. The unnecessary controversy. *Eur Heart J* 1996; 17: 1142–47.

5 Konrad Dalhoff I, Baunack AR, Ramsch KD, et al. Effect of the calcium antagonists nifedipine, nitrendipine, nimodipine and nisoldipine on oesophageal motility in man. *Eur J Clin Pharmacol* 1991; 41: 313–16.

6 Pahor M, Guralnik JM, Chrischilles EA, Wallace RB. Use of laxative medication in older persons and associations with low serum albumin. *J Am Geriatr Soc* 1994; 42: 50–56.

7 Wagenknecht LE, Furberg CD, Hammon JW, Legault C, Troost BT. Surgical bleeding: unexpected effect of a calcium antagonist. *BMJ* 1995; 310: 776–77.

8 Pahor M, Guralnik JM, Furberg CD, Carbonin PU, Havlik RJ. Risk of gastrointestinal haemorrhage with calcium antagonists in hypertensive persons over 67 years old. *Lancet* 1996; 347: 1061–65.

9 Stein G, Srivastava MK, Merker HJ, Neubert D. Effects of calcium channel blockers on the development of early rat postimplantation embryos in culture. *Arch Toxicol* 1990; 64: 623–38.

10 Crowson AN, Magro CM. Diltiazem and subacute cutaneous lupus erythematosus-like lesions. *N Engl J Med* 1995; 333: 1429.

11 Pahor M, Guralnik JM, Salive ME, Corti MC, Carbonin P, Havlik RJ. Do calcium channel blockers increase the risk of cancer? *Am J Hypertens* 1996; 9: 695–99.

12 Connor J, Sawczuk IS, Benson MC, et al. Calcium channel antagonists delay regression of androgen-dependent tissues and suppress gene activity associated with cell death. *Prostate* 1988; 13: 119–30.

13 Juntti Berggren L, Larsson O, Rorsman P, et al. Increased activity of L-type Ca^{2+} channels exposed to serum from patients with type I diabetes. *Science* 1993; 261: 86–90.

14 Ray SD, Kamendulis LM, Gurule MW, Yorkin RD, Corcoran GB. Ca^{2+} antagonists inhibit DNA fragmentation and toxic cell death induced by acetaminophen. *FASEB J* 1993; 7: 453–63.

15 Carson DA, Ribeiro JM. Apoptosis and disease. *Lancet* 1993; 341: 1251–54.

16 Trump BF, Berezesky IK. Calcium-mediated cell injury and cell death. *FASEB J* 1995; 9: 219–28.

17 Martin SJ, Green DR. Apoptosis and cancer: the failure of controls on cell death and cell survival. *Crit Rev Oncol Hematol* 1995; 18: 137–53.

18 Whitfield JF. Calcium signals and cancer. *Crit Rev Oncog* 1992; 3: 55–90.

19 Garland C, Shekelle RB, Barrett-Connor E, Criqui MH, Rossof AH, Paul O. Dietary vitamin D and calcium and risk of colorectal cancer: a 19-year prospective study in men. *Lancet* 1985; i: 307–09.

20 Cornoni-Huntley J, Ostfeld AM, Taylor JO, et al. Established populations for epidemic studies of the elderly: study design and methodology. *Aging Clin Exp Res* 1993; 5: 27–37.

21 Stampfer MJ, Willett WC, Speizer FE, Dysert DC. Test of the National Death Index. *Am J Epidemiol* 1984; 119: 837–39.

22 Fisher ES, Whaley FS, Krushat WM, et al. The accuracy of Medicare's hospital claims data: progress has been made, but problems remain. *Am J Public Hlth* 1992; 82: 243–48.

23 SEER cancer statistics review, 1973–1991: tables and graphs, National Cancer Institute. NIH publication No 94-2789. Bethesda, MD: NIH publication no 94-2789, 1994.

24 Cohen J. Weighted kappa: nominal scale agreement with provision for scaled disagreement or partial credit. *Psychol Bull* 1968; 70: 213–20.

25 Psaty BM, Lee M, Savage PJ, Rutan GH, German PS, Lyles M. Assessing the use of medications in the elderly: methods and initial experience in the Cardiovascular Health Study. *J Clin Epidemiol* 1992; 45: 638–92.

26 Pahor M, Chrischilles EA, Guralnik JM, Brown SL, Wallace RB, Carbonin PU. Drug data coding and analysis in epidemiologic studies. *Eur J Epidemiol* 1994; 10: 405–11.

27 Rose GA, Blackburn H, Gillum RF, Prineas RJ. Annex 6—London school of hygiene cardiovascular questionnaire. In: World Health Organisaton. Cardiovascular survey methods, 2nd edn. Geneva: WHO, 1982: 162–65.

28 Katz S, Ford AB, Moskowitz RW, Jackson BA, Jaffe MW. Studies of illness in the aged. The index of ADL: a standardized measure of biological and psychosocial function. *JAMA* 1963; 185: 94–99.

29 Rosow I, Breslau N. A Guttman health scale for the aged. *J Gerontol* 1966; 21: 556–59.

30 Hypertension Detection and Follow-up Program Cooperative Group. Blood pressure studies in 14 communities; a two-stage screen for hypertension. *JAMA* 1977; 237: 2385–91.

31 Tenniswood MP, Guenette RS, Lakins J, Mooibroek M, Wong P, Welsh JE. Active cell death in hormone-dependent tissues. *Cancer Metastasis Rev* 1992; 11: 197–220.

32 Batra S, Popper LD, Hartley-Asp B. Effect of calcium and calcium antagonists on 45Ca influx and cellular growth of human prostatic tumor cells. *Prostate* 1991; 19: 299–311.

33 Raynor WJ, Shekelle RB, Rossof AH, Maliza M, Paul O. High blood pressure and 17-year cancer mortality in the Western Electric Health Study. *Am J Epidemiol* 1981; 118: 371–77.

34 Dyer AR, Stamler J, Berkson DM, Lindberg HA, Stevens E. High blood pressure: a risk factor for cancer mortality? *Lancet* 1975; i: 1051–56.

35 Furberg CD, Psaty BM. Calcium antagonists: antagonists or protagonists of mortality in elderly hypertensives? *J Am Geriatr Soc* 1995; 43: 1309–10.

36 Yusuf S. Calcium antagonists in coronary artery disease and hypertension. Time for reevaluation? *Circulation* 1995; 92: 1079–82.

Session 4 – Harm & searching the primary literature

Citation:

Are the results of this harm study valid?

Were there clearly defined groups of patients, similar in all important ways other than exposure to the treatment or other cause?

Were treatment exposures and clinical outcomes measured the same way in both groups, e.g. was the assessment of outcomes either objective (death) or blinded to exposure?

Was the follow up of study patients complete and long enough?

Do the results satisfy some 'diagnostic tests for causation'?

- Is it clear that the exposure preceded the onset of the outcome?

- Is there a dose-response gradient?

- Is there positive evidence from a 'dechallenge–rechallenge' study?

- Is the association consistent from study to study?

- Does the association make biological sense?

Are the valid results from this harm study important?

		Adverse Outcome		Totals
		Present (case)	Absent (control)	
Exposed to the Treatment	Yes (cohort)	a	b	a+b
	No (cohort)	c	d	c+d
	Totals	a+c	b+d	a+b+c+d

In a randomised trial or cohort study: relative risk = RR = [a/(a+b)]/[c/(c+d)]
In a case-control study: odds ratio (or Relative odds) = OR = ad/bc
In this study:

Should these valid, potentially important results of a critical appraisal about a harmful treatment change the treatment of your patient?

Can the study results be extrapolated to your patient?

What are your patient's risks of the adverse outcome?
To calculate the NNH[1] for any odds ratio (OR) and
your patient's expected event rate for this adverse
event if they were **not** exposed to this treatment (PEER):

$$NNH = \frac{PEER\ (OR - 1) + 1}{PEER\ (OR - 1) \times (1 - PEER)}$$

What are your patient's preferences, concerns and
expectations from this treatment?

What alternative treatments are available?

Additional notes

[1] The number of patients you need to treat to harm one of them.

Citation: Pahor M *et al.* (1996) Calcium-channel blockade and incidence of cancer in aged populations. *Lancet.* **348**: 493–97 (see also pp 487–9 and 541–2).

Are the results of this harm study valid?

Were there clearly defined groups of patients, similar in all important ways other than exposure to the treatment or other cause?	**Clearly defined, but heterogeneous. Exposed individuals different from non-exposed – more diabetes and cardiovascular disease, disability, hospitalisation, but lower diastolic pressure – but both groups cancer-free at the start of the study.**
Were treatment exposures and clinical outcomes measured the same way in both groups, e.g. was the assessment of outcomes either objective (death) or blinded to exposure)?	**Yes. Asked to show their medications, and clinical outcomes measured the same way in both groups.**
Was the follow-up of study patients complete and long enough?	**Averaged 3.7 years and long enough to show a positive relationship between CCBs and cancer. But there were only 47 cancers in 1549 person-years of CCB taking.**

Do the results satisfy some 'diagnostic tests for causation'?

• Is it clear that the exposure preceded the onset of the outcome?	**Probably – excluded everyone with known cancer at the start (still may have been some smouldering).**
• Is there a dose-response gradient?	**Yes – Figure 2.**
• Is there positive evidence from a 'dechallenge–rechallenge' study?	**No.**
• Is the association consistent from study to study?	**No.**
• Does the association make biological sense?	**Whether interference with apoptotic destruction of cancer cells is sensible is hotly debated.**

BUT: was this a previously generated hypothesis, or was it one of several analyses carried out on a large data set of drugs and diseases? (We have written to the authors about this and Dr. Pahor has informed us that this hypotheses was generated prior to the study onset.)

Are the valid results from this harm study important?

		Adverse Outcome		Totals
		Present (case)	Absent (control)	
Exposed to the Treatment	Yes (cohort)	3.03% a	b	a+b
	No (cohort)	c 2.17%	d	c+d
	Totals	a+c	b+d	a+b+c+d

In this study: relative risk = RR = 3.03%/2.17% = 1.4 (P = 0.032) (and when adjusted for several baseline differences, RR ROSE (!) to 1.7 (P = 0.0005)).

Should these valid, potentially important results of a critical appraisal about a harmful treatment change the treatment of your patient?

Can the study results be extrapolated to your patient?

Depends on whether you believe them. If you do believe them, they can be extrapolated to your patient.

What are your patient's risks of the adverse outcome? To calculate the NNH[1] for any odds ratio (OR) and your patient's expected event rate for this adverse event if they were **not** exposed to this treatment (PEER):

$$NNH = \frac{PEER\,(OR - 1) + 1}{PEER\,(OR - 1) \times (1 - PEER)}$$

If we assume our patient is like the average individual in this study (the hazard ratios are like odds ratios and don't differ in important ways between subgroups), then his absolute risk increase in cancer over 3.7 years is 3.03% − 2.17% = 0.86% = and 1/0.86% gives an NNH of 116.

What are your patient's preferences, concerns and expectations from this treatment?

Need to be determined.

What alternative treatments are available?

Lots of alternative treatments available for his hypertension (thiazides, beta-blockers). They have their own side-effects but are not reputed to cause cancer.

Additional notes

1 Other case-control and cohort studies vary in their conclusions about CCB risks, and a meta-analysis is awaited.

Until it is sorted out, you could describe NNHs (and possible NNHs) for alternative antihypertensive regimens with your patient and the two of you could collaborate in deciding on the most appropriate one for him.

[1] The number of patients you need to treat to harm one of them.

HYPERTENSION – CALCIUM-CHANNEL BLOCKERS MAY CAUSE CANCER

Appraised by David Sackett 1996.
Expiry date: 2000.

Clinical Bottom Line

1 Until this gets sorted out properly, if your patient's problem could be treated as well by some alternative drug, e.g. hypertension, it would be prudent to avoid using calcium-channel agents.

2 If this result is true, the NNH to cause one additional cancer from taking CCBs for 3.7 years is 116.

Citation

Pahor M *et al.* (1996) Calcium-channel blockade and incidence of cancer in aged populations. *Lancet.* **348:** 493–97 (also see 487–9 and 541–2).

Clinical Question

In patients taking calcium antagonists for hypertension, are they at increased risk of cancer?

Search terms

From the newspaper headline or from MEDLINE using 'calcium antagonists' and 'cancer'.

The Study

Total or stratified random samples (>80% response rate) of 65+ year old men and women in three sites in the USA. They showed their meds, were interviewed for 90 minutes and had their blood pressure, height and weight measured. Anyone with cancer in the previous three years or on any cancer Rx was excluded and 94% of the remainder were followed for an average of 3.7 years by follow-up interview, hospital discharge information and the national death registry for the occurrence of new cancers.

The Evidence

		Late cancer		Totals
		Present	**Absent**	
Exposed to calcium channel blockers	Yes (cohort)	3.03% a	b	a+b
	No (cohort)	2.17% c	d	c+d
	Totals	a+c	b+d	a+b+c+d

Relative risk = RR = 3.03%/2.17% = 1.4 (P = 0.032) (and when adjusted for several baseline differences, RR ROSE (!) to 1.7 (P = 0.0005)).

Comments

1 Individuals on CCBs had more cardiovascular disease, diabetes, disability, and hospitalisations but lower diastolic blood pressure. But when they adjusted for all these baseline differences, the RR rose rather than fell, suggesting that bias from confounding (of cancer risk and CCB use) of these characteristics could not explain these results.

2 There was a dose-response gradient.

3 The difference in risk by type of CCB was impressive but not statistically significant (RR 2 for verapamil; 1.5 for nifedipine; 0.94 for diltiazem).

4 Only 47 events in CCB takers and spread over all sorts of different cancers.

5 The proposed mechanism (interference with the apoptotic destruction of cancer cells) dismissed by commentators.

6 Other studies of CCBs and mortality go both ways (they are bad or have no effect), and some authors of the former have received anonymous death threats.

PART A

Critical appraisal of a systematic review about stroke units

You are referred a 75-year old man with a stroke who had been admitted one day previously to general medicine. He has left-sided weakness and has difficulty with ambulating, bathing, feeding and dressing himself. He has hypertension which is well controlled with a diuretic. He is otherwise well and you decide to transfer him to a stroke unit. His family is concerned because they live close to the hospital where he is currently an inpatient and want to know why he needs to be transferred to a stroke unit of a different hospital and why he can't stay on the general medicine ward. You (with them) formulate the question: 'In a patient with a stroke, does admission to a stroke unit decrease the risk of death and dependency?'

You search *Best Evidence* using the terms 'stroke unit' and 'death' and find a promising systematic review. The abstract and commentary look helpful and you decide to retrieve the complete article: *BMJ.* (1997) **314:** 1151–9.

Read the systematic review and decide:

1 Is the evidence from this systematic review valid?
2 Is this valid evidence from this systematic review important?
3 Can you apply this valid and important evidence from this systematic review in caring for your patient?

If you want to read some strategies for answering these sorts of questions, you could have a look at pp 97–9, 140–1 and 166–72 in *Evidence-based Medicine.*

PART B

Searching for evidence in the Cochrane Library

We will show you how to search the Cochrane Library, an electronic database of systematic reviews done by the Cochrane Collaboration, abstracts of other systematic reviews from the world literature, citations from several hundred thousand randomised trials and information about the Cochrane Collaboration.

To help us organise your presentations for Sessions 6 and 7, please complete and hand in the form on the next page.

CASE
PRESENTATION

My tentative clinical question:

My name: _____

Contact address: _____

Contact phone number: _____

Bleep: _____

E-mail: _____

Papers

Collaborative systematic review of the randomised trials of organised inpatient (stroke unit) care after stroke

Stroke Unit Trialists' Collaboration

Abstract

Objectives: To define the characteristics and determine the effectiveness of organised inpatient (stroke unit) care compared with conventional care in reducing death, dependency, and the requirement for long term institutional care after stroke.

Design: Systematic review of all randomised trials which compared organised inpatient stroke care with the contemporary conventional care. Specialist stroke unit interventions were defined as either a ward or team exclusively managing stroke (dedicated stroke unit) or a ward or team specialising in the management of disabling illnesses, which include stroke (mixed assessment/rehabilitation unit). Conventional care was usually provided in a general medical ward.

Setting: 19 trials (of which three had two treatment arms). 12 trials randomised a total of 2060 patients to a dedicated stroke unit or a general medical ward, six trials (647 patients) compared a mixed assessment/rehabilitation unit with a general medical ward, and four trials (542 patients) compared a dedicated stroke unit with a mixed assessment/rehabilitation unit.

Main outcome measures: Death, institutionalisation, and dependency.

Results: Organised inpatient (stroke unit) care, when compared with conventional care, was best characterised by coordinated multidisciplinary rehabilitation, programmes of education and training in stroke, and specialisation of medical and nursing staff. The stroke unit care was usually housed in a geographically discrete ward. Stroke unit care was associated with a long term (median one year follow up) reduction of death (odds ratio 0.83, 95% confidence interval 0.69 to 0.98; P < 0.05) and of the combined poor outcomes of death or dependency (0.69, 0.59 to 0.82; P < 0.0001) and death or institutionalisation (0.75, 0.65 to 0.87; P < 0.0001). Beneficial effects were independent of patients' age, sex, or stroke severity and of variations in stroke unit organisation. Length of stay in a hospital or institution was reduced by 8% (95% confidence interval 3% to 13%) compared with conventional care but there was considerable heterogeneity of results.

Conclusions: Organised stroke unit care resulted in long term reductions in death, dependency, and the need for institutional care. The observed benefits were not restricted to any particular subgroup of patients or model of stroke unit care. No systematic increase in the use of resources (in terms of length of stay) was apparent.

Stroke Unit Trialists' Collaboration

A list of collaborators is given at the end of the article.

Correspondence to: Dr Peter Langhorne, Academic Section of Geriatric Medicine, Royal Infirmary, Glasgow G4 0SF

BMJ 1997;314:1151–9

Introduction

The role of organised (stroke unit) care in managing inpatients with stroke has been controversial for over 30 years.[1] The controversy arises because the moderate benefits that might be anticipated with stroke unit care can be reliably detected (or refuted) only with a very large randomised trial or a proper overview of the available small randomised trials. Evaluation of stroke unit care raises particular problems because of the complex and heterogeneous nature of the intervention and its potential interaction with other aspects of care. Even a prospective multicentre randomised trial could not guarantee a uniform intervention because the service characteristics would inevitably vary between centres.

Systematic review (including meta-analysis) methods combine the available evidence from randomised trials to draw more reliable and generalisable conclusions.[2] Our review of randomised trials available up to October 1993 indicated that specialist stroke unit care may reduce death and institutionalisation after stroke.[3] However, we did not have detailed descriptions of service organisation or detailed information on many outcomes or subgroups of interest and substantial new information has now become available from several recently completed randomised trials.

We conducted a further systematic review to determine whether the apparent benefits of organised stroke unit care were confirmed in a more extensive and updated analysis, examine outcomes in addition to death and institutionalisation, examine the effects in subgroups of stroke patients and with various models of specialist stroke unit care, provide a detailed description of stroke unit and control interventions, and identify the features associated with an improved outcome. To meet these objectives a collaborative review group was formed which included trialists from the available randomised controlled trials.

Methods

We aimed to compare any system of organised inpatient stroke care with the less organised conventional practice. We therefore included all prospective trials that used some form of randomisation to allocate patients to an organised stroke unit or conventional care, usually in general medical wards. Trials were included if treatment allocation was carried out on a strictly random basis or a quasi-randomised procedure (such as date of admission). We excluded studies which compared specific therapies within an organised stroke care setting.

Our objectives were to examine the effect of organised stroke unit care on the outcomes of death, dependency, and the requirement for institutional care (all recorded at the end of scheduled follow up in an intention to treat analysis).

Identification of trials

We identified relevant research reports up to December 1995 using several approaches.[3] In summary, we carried out systematic hand searches of 22 core neurology and stroke journals and five Japanese journals and systematic searches of Index Medicus, Medline, and dissertation abstracts. We searched the reference lists of trials, review articles, and textbooks; Current Contents; and the proceedings of 43 recent conferences on neurology, geriatric medicine, and rehabilitation. Further information was obtained by talking to colleagues and publicising our preliminary findings at stroke conferences in the United Kingdom, Scandinavia, Germany, Switzerland, Spain, Canada, and South America.

Definition of interventions

Although the primary question was whether organised inpatient stroke care could improve outcomes compared with contemporary conventional care, we divided the organisation of service into one of the following three predefined groups to reflect the heterogeneity of services.

Dedicated stroke unit—A service provided by a discrete stroke ward or stroke team working exclusively in the care of stroke patients. This category included acute (intensive) stroke units, which accept patients acutely but discharge early (usually within seven days); rehabilitation stroke units, which accept patients after a minimum delay of seven days and focus on rehabilitation; and combined acute/rehabilitation units, which accept patients acutely but also provides rehabilitation for at least several weeks. Both the rehabilitation unit and combined acute/rehabilitation unit models offered prolonged periods of rehabilitation.

Mixed assessment/rehabilitation unit—A ward or team which has an interest and expertise in the assessment and rehabilitation of disabling illness but does not exclusively manage stroke patients.

General medical wards—A service provided in wards which focus on the management of acutely ill general medical patients but not on their subsequent rehabilitation. In most trials this formed the control group.

Definition of outcome measures

The primary analyses examined death, dependency, and the requirement for institutional care at the end of scheduled follow up. Dependency was categorised into two groups where independent was taken to mean that an individual did not require physical assistance for transfers, mobility, dressing, feeding, or toileting.

Individuals who failed any of these criteria were considered dependent. The criteria for independence were roughly equivalent to a Rankin score of 0-2 or a Barthel score of > 18/20.[4] The requirement for long term institutional care was taken as meaning care in a residential home, nursing home, or hospital at the end of the rehabilitation period. Length of stay in a hospital or institution was also recorded.

Data from contributing trials

The principal investigators of all the trials that fulfilled the criteria of the overview were invited to join the Stroke Unit Trialists' Collaboration. All who could be contacted agreed to join. They were asked to provide details of their trial design, including the method of treatment allocation, selection criteria, characteristics of patients, details of service organisation, duration of interventions, duration of follow up, numbers in each outcome group, and additional services after discharge from hospital. The survey of trial characteristics included a structured interview with the trial coordinator, carried out by a single interviewer (PL), which focused on aspects of the structure, staffing, organisation, selection criteria, and procedures and practices within the stroke unit and control settings. For the three trials for which a coordinator could not be contacted we have used the best available published information.

Wherever possible we obtained basic outcome data at the end of scheduled follow up for all patients randomised (to permit an intention to treat analysis). Most trials could be analysed on this basis, at least for the outcomes of death and death or requiring institutional care. Those trials with incomplete follow up were analysed with the assumption that patients lost to follow up were alive and living at home. The implications of these assumptions were explored in a sensitivity analysis.

Outcome information was also sought for subgroups of patients based on age, sex, and stroke severity. Severity of stroke at the time of randomisation was defined by patients' initial dependency (within the first week after stroke). Where randomisation was carried out at different times after stroke, initial dependency was inferred from published information on the expected rate of functional recovery[5]:

Mild stroke—Patient can transfer and walk (with or without assistance) during the first week after the stroke. This is roughly equivalent to a Barthel score of > 10/20 (Rankin score 0-3) within one week of the stroke or > 13/20 (0-3) by two weeks after the stroke.

Moderate stroke—Patient is conscious and has sitting balance but is unable to stand or walk during the first week after stroke.

Severe stroke—Patient has reduced consciousness or no sitting balance, or both, during the first week after stroke; equivalent to a Barthel score of < 3/20 (Rankin 5) within one week or < 4/20 (5) by two weeks.

Although the inaccuracies inherent in this process are likely to have resulted in some misclassification of patients, the criteria were applied equally to stroke unit and control patients. Most trials used exclusion criteria such that patients with the mildest and severest strokes would be excluded.

We sought individual patient data for all trials, but unfortunately insufficient data were available to permit

1152

Table 1 Characteristics of trials contributing data to the review

Trial	Participants	Comparison groups	Outcomes	Notes
Birmingham[10]	Stroke patients within 2 weeks of a stroke	Intensive rehabilitation in rehabilitation centre MARU (n=29) v normal care in general wards (n=23)	Death and dependency at the end of follow up (6-8 months)	Timing of outcomes not clear. Intervention not defined. 3 control patients lost to follow up
Dover[11]	Stroke patients within 9 weeks (most within 3 weeks of a stroke)	DSU in stroke rehabilitation ward (n=116) v geriatric medicine MARU (n=28) or GMW (n=89)	Death, Rankin score, place of residence, length of hospital stay up to 1 year after stroke	Minor randomisation imbalance. Numbers differ slightly from published report following reanalysis of original data. 2 Control patients lost to follow up
Edinburgh[12]	Acute stroke patients (moderate severity) within 7 days of stroke	DSU in stroke rehabilitation ward (n=155) v GMW (n=156)	Death, dependency, place of residence, length of hospital stay up to 1 year after stroke	6 Intervention and 10 control lost to follow up
Goteborg-Ostra[13]	Acute stroke patients within 7 days after stroke	Combined acute and rehabilitation DSU within general medical service (n=215) v conventional care in GMW (n=202)	Death, Barthel score, place of residence, length of hospital stay	Not yet published
Goteborg-Sahlgren[14]	Acute stroke patients within 7 days after stroke	Combined acute and rehabilitation DSU v conventional care in GMW	Death, Barthel score, place of residence, patient satisfaction, length of hospital stay up to 1 year	Not yet published
Helsinki[15]	Acute stroke patients, over 65 years age (within 7 days after stroke)	MARU in neurology ward (n=121) v conventional care in GMW (n=122)	Death, Barthel and Rankin scores, length of hospital stay up to 1 year	Intention to treat (on treatment analysis gave less conservative result)
Illinois[16]	Stroke patients up to 1 year after stroke	MARU in rehabilitation service (n=56) v GMW (n=35) which had some specialist nursing input	Functional status and place of residence at end of follow up	Poor definition of services. No deaths reported. 3:2 allocation to intervention:control
Kuopio[17]	Stroke patients (at 1 week after stroke) able to tolerate intensive rehabilitation	DSU in neurological service (n=50) v GMW (n=45)	Death, ADL score, place of residence, duration of hospital stay up to 1 year	Most patients screened failed to meet inclusion criteria for the trial
Montreal[18]	Acute stroke patients with 7 days of a stroke	DSU (mobile stroke team; n=65) v conventional care in GMW (n=65)	Death, Barthel score, place of residence, length of initial hospital stay up to 6 weeks after stroke	Short follow up period. One intervention patient and 3 controls lost to follow up
New York[19]	Stroke patients up to 2 months after stroke	MARU in rehabilitation centre (n=42) v general wards (n=40) with some specialist nursing input	Functional status and place of residence at end of follow up (about 1 year)	No deaths reported. Minor anomaly in published data table
Newcastle[20]	Acute stroke patients (within 3 days after stroke)	MARU in geriatric medicine department (n=33) v GMW (n=33)	Death, Barthel and Rankin scores, place of residence, length of hospital stay up to 6 months after stroke	Most patients screened did not meet trial inclusion criteria
Nottingham[21]	Stroke patients 2 weeks after stroke	DSU (stroke rehabilitation ward) in geriatric medicine department (n=176) v MARU in geriatric medicine department (n=63) or GMW (n=76)	Death, Barthel score, place of residence, length of hospital stay up to 6 months after stroke	Some crossover from GMW to geriatric medicine; 5:4 allocation to intervention:control. 3 Intervention patients and 4 controls lost to follow up
Orpington (1993)[22]	Stroke patients at 2 weeks after stroke	DSU (stroke rehabilitation ward) in geriatric medicine department (n=124) v MARU in geriatric medicine department (n=73) or GMW (n=48)	Death, Barthel score, place of residence, length of hospital stay at end of follow up	Variable duration of follow up
Orpington (1995)[23]	Stroke patients who have a poor prognosis at 2 weeks after stroke	DSU (stroke rehabilitation ward) in geriatric medicine department (n=36) v GMW (n=37)	Death, Barthel score, place of residence, length of hospital stay at end of follow up	Variable duration of follow up. Two control patients lost to follow up
Perth[24]	Acute stroke patients within 7 days after stroke	Combined acute and rehabilitation DSU in neurology department (n=28) v GMW (n=30)	Death, Barthel score, place of residence, length of hospital stay up to 6 months after stroke	Most patients screened did not enter trial
Tampere[25]	Acute stroke patients within 7 days after stroke (usually earlier)	Acute, intensive DSU in neurology department (n=98) v MARU in a neurology department (n=113)	Death, Rankin score, place of residence, length of hospital stay up to 1 year after stroke	Short duration (1 week) in DSU before transfer to conventional service
Trondheim[26]	Acute stroke patients within 7 days (usually within 24 hours) after stroke	Combined acute and rehabilitation DSU (n=110) v GMW (n=110)	Death, Barthel score, place of residence, length of stay in hospital or institution up to 1 year	Intention to treat data used
Umea[27]	Acute stroke patients within 7 days of stroke	Combined acute rehabilitation DSU (n=110) v GMW (n=183)	Death, functional status, place of residence, length of initial hospital stay up to 1 year after stroke	Quasi-randomised. Treatment allocation according to bed availability
Uppsala[28]	Stroke patients admitted to general medical wards within 3 days of stroke	MARU (organised care within GMW; n=60) v conventional care in GMW (n=52)	Death, ADL score, place of residence, length of stay in acute hospital up to 1 year after stroke	Quasi-randomised. Treatment allocation according to admission rota

Unless otherwise stated, all trials are randomised controlled with balanced allocation to intervention and control groups.
DSU=Dedicated stroke unit (managing stoke patients only), MARU=Mixed assessment/rehabilitation unit (managing other disabling illness as well as stroke), GMW=General medical ward (general medical ward).

a comprehensive individual patient data analysis. The available data were, however, used to cross check the results obtained as summary data.

Statistical methods

Dichotomous outcomes
The formal statistical methods used to combine the results from different trials have been described elsewhere.[6] Within each trial the standard quantity "observed minus expected" (together with its variance) was calculated for the numbers of events among patients allocated to treatment groups. The grand totals of the individual observed minus expected values and of their

variance were used to calculate P values and odds ratios.[6] The odds ratio gives the odds of an unfavourable outcome among patients in the treated groups compared with control patients stratified by trial.

This approach (fixed effects model) assumes that each trial result is sufficiently similar to the other results to differ only by chance. Where this is not the case, statistical heterogeneity exists. When heterogeneity was found the sources were explored[7] and results confirmed by a random effects model analysis.[8]

Continuous variables
Continuous variable data (length of stay) were analysed as the weighted mean difference—that is, the difference

Table 2 Frequency of various characteristics within organised (stroke unit) care and conventional care settings. Values are numbers (percentages) of arms of trials with available data

Characteristics	Organised care	Conventional care	P value*
Disciplines routinely involved in stroke care:			
Medical	22/22 (100)	18/18 (100)	NS
Nursing	22/22 (100)	18/18 (100)	NS
Physiotherapy	22/22 (100)	18/18 (100)	NS
Occupational therapy	21/22 (95)	17/18 (94)	NS
Speech therapy	18/19 (81)	15/18 (83)	NS
Social work	18/19 (81)	17/18 (94)	NS
Coordination of rehabilitation:			
Multidisciplinary team care (weekly meetings)	19 /19 (100)	4/19 (21)	<0.0001
Nursing integrated with multidisciplinary team	19/19 (100)	4/19 (21)	<0.0001
Carers routinely involved in rehabilitation	17/19 (89)	2/19 (11)	<0.0001
Carers routinely attend multidisciplinary team meetings	6/18 (33)	0/18 (0)	0.01
Education and training:			
Routine information provision to carers	17/19 (89)	2/19 (11)	<0.0001
Regular staff training	17 /20(85)	1/20 (5)	<0.0001
Specialisation of staff:			
Nursing interest in rehabilitation	18/19 (95)	4/21 (21)	<0.0001
Physician interest in stroke	14/19 (74)	2/19 (11)	0.0001
Nursing interest in stroke	14/19 (74)	2/19 (11)	0.0001
Physician interest in rehabilitation	13/21 (62)	3/21 (14)	0.002
Comprehensiveness of rehabilitation input:			
Increased proportion of patients receive physiotherapy or occupational therapy	9/17 (53)	0/17 (0)	0.0005
Earlier onset of physiotherapy or occupational therapy	7/20 (35)	0/19 (0)	0.004
Medical investigation/treatment protocol	5/19 (26)	0/20 (0)	0.02
Intensity of rehabilitaion input:			
More intensive physiotherapy or occupational therapy	8/19 (42)	2/18 (11)	0.03
Enhanced nurse:patient ratio	5/18 (28)	1/17 (6)	NS

*P values were calculated with Fisher's exact test (NS denotes P>0.05)

between mean values in the treatment and control groups of individual trials and the mean difference weighted for trial size for groups of trials.[9] The 95% confidence intervals of the weighted mean difference were calculated by using the mean and standard deviation data from the individual trials. Because the length of stay was calculated in different ways for different trials, results were calculated from both absolute values (days) and relative change in length of stay (expressed as a percentage of the length of stay in the control group).

Absolute outcomes

Absolute outcome rates, expressed as the proportion of patients in each outcome group are less statistically robust but more clinically meaningful than relative changes in outcomes. The number needed to treat to prevent one adverse outcome was calculated as the reciprocal of the difference in absolute outcome rates between the treatment and control groups.

Results

A total of 19 trials were identified by December 1995.[10-28] Seventeen were formally randomised by using random numbers or sequentially numbered sealed envelopes and two used informal procedures based on bed availability[27] or a strict admission rota.[28] These two trials were evaluated separately to exclude significant bias in the conclusions.

Of the 19 trials identified, one has not yet been completed[14] while the remaining 18 contained a total of 3249 patients. Eleven trials (2060 patients)

compared a dedicated stroke unit with a general medical ward, six (647 patients) compared a mixed assessment/rehabilitation unit with a general medical ward, and four (542 patients) compared a dedicated stroke unit with a mixed assessment/rehabilitation unit (table 1). The total number of comparisons is greater than the number of trials because in three trials patients could be randomised to one of two conventional care groups; two of these trials[21 22] used a stratified randomisation procedure and one[11] did not.

Detailed descriptive information on service characteristics could not be obtained by structured interview for only three trials.[10 16 19] In 18 trials stroke unit care included rehabilitation lasting several weeks if required; 10 of these units admitted patients acutely and eight after a delay of one to two weeks. Only one trial evaluated an acute stroke unit with no continuing rehabilitation.[25]

In 17 of the trials the organised care was provided in a geographically discrete ward; two trials examined peripatetic systems of care.[18 28] Table 2 summarises the service comparisons within the trials. Stroke unit interventions were more likely to be reported to include coordinated multidisciplinary rehabilitation, staff with a specialist interest in stroke or rehabilitation, and regular programmes of education and training. Several factors indicating a more intensive or more comprehensive input of care were less significantly associated with stroke unit care.

Summary data on death, placement, and dependency at the end of scheduled follow up were available for 21, 20, and 20 comparisons respectively. In one trial the number of dependent patients had to be calculated from the mean and standard deviation Barthel score results.[18] Six trials had minor omissions of data during follow up (total 10 stroke unit patients and 25 controls).[10-12 18 25 27] As these patients were assumed to be alive and living at home, this may have introduced a minor basis in favour of the control group.

Within the stroke unit group 340/1626 (20.9%) patients were dead at the end of follow up (median one year after stroke), 304/1597 (19.0%) were in institutional care, and 519/1409 (36.8%) were dependent. The corresponding figures for controls were 413/1623 (25.4%) dead, 344/1600 (21.5%) in institutional care, and 543/1421 (38.2%)dependent. The minor variation in the denominator is due to placement and dependency data each being unavailable for one trial.

Death only

Figure 1 shows the odds of death by the end of scheduled follow up in different forms of stroke unit versus conventional care. The summary result (odds ratio 0.82, 95% confidence interval 0.69 to 0.98; P<0.05) was not complicated by significant heterogeneity between trials (χ^2= 13.6, df= 18; P>0.2). There was no detectable variation between the treatment effects in the three subgroup comparisons in figure 1. The odds of death was essentially unchanged if the analysis was restricted to trials where scheduled follow up was continued for a fixed period of six months or one year (0.84, 0.70 to 1.04; P<0.1).[11 12 15 17 19 20 21 24-28] The exclusion of two trials with an informal randomisation procedure[27 28] did not affect the conclusions (0.81, 0.67 to 0.98; P<0.05).

BMJ VOLUME 314   19 APRIL 1997

Death or institutionalisation

The second outcome examined (fig 2) was the odds of death or requiring institutional care at the end of follow up (median one year after stroke). The summary result (0.75, 0.65 to 0.87; P<0.0001) was highly significant but some heterogeneity existed between trials ($\chi^2 = 25.9$, df = 19; P = 0.1). Reanalysis of the results with a random effects model produced similar results (0.74, 0.62 to 0.89; P<0.0001). The observed heterogeneity was largely attributable to the five trials that had a short (less than six weeks) or variable period of follow up ($\chi^2 = 14$, df = 4; P<0.01).[13 16 18 22 23] Trials with a fixed follow up period showed a significant reduction in death or institutionalisation (0.76, 0.64 to 0.90; P<0.01) with much less heterogeneity ($\chi^2 = 11.5$, df = 13; P>0.2). There was no significant variation between the treatment effects in the three subgroup comparisons. The estimate of apparent benefits was unaffected if informally randomised trials were excluded.

Death or dependency

The third outcome examined was the combined adverse outcome of being dead or dependent in activities of daily living at the end of follow up (fig 3). The overall odds ratio of being dead or dependent if given stroke unit care rather than conventional care was 0.71 (0.61 to 0.84; P<0.0001) but the summary result showed some heterogeneity ($\chi^2 = 16.1$, df = 19; P>0.2). Reanalysis with a random effects model produced similar results (0.72, 0.61 to 0.83; P<0.0001). The main source of heterogeneity seems to reflect the nature of the control group. Results were less heterogeneous ($\chi^2 = 10$, df = 12; P>0.2) and odds ratios remained significant (0.66, 0.55 to 0.79; P<0.0001) where either a dedicated stroke unit or a mixed assessment/rehabilitation ward was compared with a general medical ward. The conclusions were not altered by the exclusion of trials with a variable follow up period[10 18 22 23] or informal randomisation procedure[27 28] or where numbers of dependent patients were calculated from continuous data.[18]

The main methodological difficulties with using dependency as an outcome was the degree of blinding of the final assessment and the potential for bias if the assessor was aware of the treatment allocation. Five trials used an unequivocally blinded final assessment for all patients.[15 17 18 21 27] The odds ratio for death or dependency in that group was 0.72 (0.55 to 0.94; P<0.01).

Absolute outcome rates

The proportion of patients dead at the end of scheduled follow up was 340/1626 (20.9%) in the stroke unit group and 413/1623 (25.4%) in the controls. On this basis the number needed to treat to prevent one death is 22. Interpreting absolute outcome rates can be problematical if the baseline event rate is variable.[29] As the baseline fatality rate varied from 0-50% in individual trials the number needed to treat might be expected to range from about 10 to infinity in the different study populations.

The proportion of patients who were unable to live at home at the end of follow up was 640/1597 (40.1%) in the stroke unit group and 755/1600 (47.2%) in the controls (number needed to treat of 14). The baseline

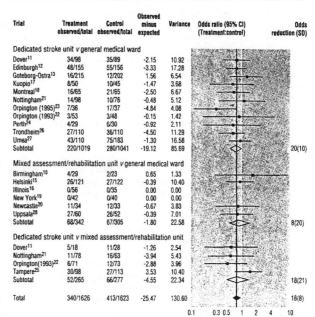

Fig 1 Odds of death occurring by end of scheduled follow up in stroke unit compared with conventional care. Odds ratios and 95% confidence intervals of individual trials are presented as a black box and horizontal line. The pooled odds ratio and 95% confidence interval for a group of trials is represented by an open diamond; the black diamond shows the pooled result for all trials. Data were not available for one trial[14]

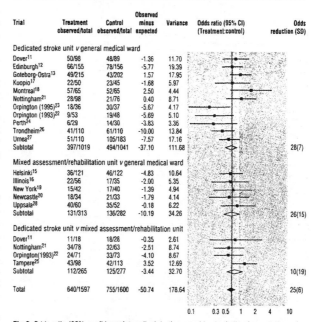

Fig 2 Odds ratio (95% confidence interval) of death or requiring institutional care at the end of scheduled follow up in patients receiving stroke unit compared with conventional care. Abbreviations and terms as for fig 1. Data were not available for two trials[10 14]

rate in individual trials ranged from 21-81% thus the number needed to treat might range from 8 to 30.

In total 843/1409 (60.0%) stroke unit patients and 944/1421 (66.4%) control patients failed to regain independence (number needed to treat of 16). With baseline rates of death or dependency of 39-100%, the range in the number needed to treat would be about 10 to 25.

Length of stay

Mean or median length of stay was available for 18 trial comparisons. Length of stay was calculated in different ways (for example, acute hospital stay, total stay in hospital or institution). Mean length of stay ranged from 13-162 days in the stroke unit groups and 14-137 days in controls. Ten trials reported a shorter length of stay in the stroke unit group[12 15 22-27] and eight a more prolonged stay.[11 13 17 18 20 21 28] The calculation of weighted mean differences in length of stay was subject to methodological limitations. Five trials reported median rather than mean length of stay[13-23] and in six trials the standard deviation was inferred from the P value or the standard deviation results from similar trials.[12 13 22 23 25 26] Overall, there was a relative reduction in length of stay in the stroke unit group of 8% (3-13%). When length of stay was calculated from absolute values (days) there was a non-significant reduction (− 0.3, 95% confidence interval − 1.8 to 1.1 days). Both the summary estimates were complicated by considerable heterogeneity which limits the extent to which general conclusions can be inferred.

Subgroup analysis

Figure 4 shows the subgroup analyses in terms of relative reduction of the combined adverse outcome of death or requiring long term institutional care. Details

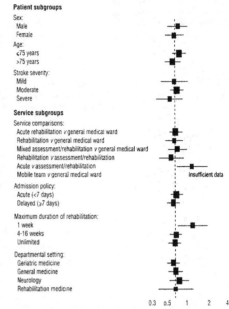

Fig 4 Analysis of patient and service characteristics on effectiveness of stroke unit care versus conventional care. Results are presented as odds ratio (95% confidence interval) of combined adverse outcome of death or requiring long term institutional care. Departmental setting refers to the medical department in which organised stroke unit care was established.

of important subgroups were available for most trials (at least 2000 patients randomised). There was no clear association of the patients' age, sex, or stroke severity with the effectiveness of organised stroke unit care. However, a relatively small number of events were observed, limiting the statistical power.

Figure 4 also outlines the relative reduction in adverse outcomes in a variety of service subgroups. Combined acute/rehabilitation stroke wards, stroke rehabilitation wards, and mixed acute/rehabilitation wards all tended to have better results than conventional care in general medical wards. There were insufficient data to comment on the acute stroke unit and roving stroke team evaluations. Benefits were apparent across units with different forms of admission policy, and within different departmental settings, and across all units which provided rehabilitation.

Publication bias

Publication bias (the selective non-reporting of trial results considered to be neutral or negative) is a potential problem for any systematic review.[30] The degree to which the conclusions of the overview would be overturned by missing neutral trials can be estimated by calculating how many randomised patients (with a similar baseline event rate as in the overview) would have to be recruited from neutral trials (odds ratio = 1.0) to render the overall result non-significant (P = 0.05). These estimates for the mortality, combined death and institutionalisation, and combined death and dependency outcomes are >500, >4000, and >6000 respectively. We also examined the distribution

Trial	Treatment observed/total	Control observed/total	Observed minus expected	Variance	Odds ratio (95% CI) (Treatment:control)	Odds reduction (SD)
Dedicated stroke unit v general medical ward						
Dover[11]	54/98	60/89	−5.74	11.16		
Edinburgh[12]	93/155	94/156	−0.20	18.70		
Kuopio[17]	31/50	31/45	−1.63	5.43		
Montreal[18]	58/65	60/65	−1.00	2.74		
Nottingham[21]	63/98	52/76	−1.77	9.65		
Orpington (1995)[23]	34/34	37/37	0.00	0.00		
Orpington (1993)[22]	38/53	39/48	−2.41	4.61		
Perth[24]	10/29	14/30	−1.80	3.62		
Trondheim[26]	54/110	81/110	−13.50	13.10		
Umea[27]	52/110	102/183	−5.82	17.19		
Subtotal	487/802	570/839	−33.86	86.20		32(8)
Mixed assessment/rehabilitation unit v general medical ward						
Birmingham[10]	8/29	9/23	−1.48	2.88		
Helsinki[15]	47/121	65/122	−8.77	15.13		
Illinois[16]	20/56	17/35	−2.77	5.25		
New York[19]	23/42	23/40	−0.56	5.11		
Newcastle[20]	26/34	28/33	−1.40	2.66		
Uppsala[28]	45/60	41/52	−1.07	5.01		
Subtotal	169/342	183/305	−16.05	36.07		36(12)
Dedicated stroke unit v mixed assessment/rehabilitation unit						
Dover[11]	11/18	19/28	−0.74	2.54		
Nottingham[21]	60/78	48/63	−0.26	6.29		
Orpington(1993)[22]	63/71	69/73	−2.08	2.77		
Tampere[25]	53/98	55/113	2.84	13.18		
Subtotal	187/265	191/277	−0.27	24.78		−1(25)
Total	843/1409	944/1421	−49.65	147.04		29(7)

0.1   0.3 0.5   1   2   4   10

Fig 3 Odds of death or dependency at the end of scheduled follow up with stroke unit compared with conventional care. Abbreviations and terms as for fig 1. Data were not available for two trials[13 14]

---

of individual trial results in relation to the trial size in a funnel plot.[30] No obvious deficiency of small, negative trials was observed.

Finally we examined the prospective sample of ongoing trials which were identified and recruited before any results were known.[15 21-25] This included 1558 patients and the odds ratio for the combined outcome of death or institutionalisation was 0.73 (95% confidence interval 0.63 to 0.84; P < 0.001).

Discussion

Systematic reviews (including meta-analysis) provide a method for examining the results of randomised trials of interventions which may have modest but clinically important effects.[2] There are several potential advantages in having a collaborative review approach, where representatives from each of the original trials are recruited into the study group. Firstly, the network of trialists recruited often have valuable information about unpublished or unfinished randomised trials, thus reducing the risk of publication bias. Secondly, the collaborative approach can allow standardised descriptions of intervention characteristics which would otherwise be reported in a manner which is not sufficiently detailed, standard, or consistent between trials. Thirdly, the collaborative review approach allows the collection of standardised subgroup and outcome information. Finally, interpretation of overviews of complex interventions can be problematical unless one can call on the collective experience and data of the trialists who are aware of the context and practical constraints within which the original randomised trials operated. Overviews based on a reanalysis of individual patient data provide the "gold standard" meta-analysis.[31] We were not able to pursue this approach because these data were not available for a substantial number of trials. However, we have been able to provide standard data sets and provide much more information than could be obtained from published data alone.

Stroke unit characteristics
Our results indicate that the benefits of organised stroke unit care, as opposed to conventional care, are not clearly due to the structure, departmental setting, staff mix, or the amount of medical, nursing, and therapy input available. The most distinctive features seem to be those of organisation (coordinated multidisciplinary team care, nursing integration with multidisciplinary care, and involvement of carers in the rehabilitation process), specialisation (medical and nursing interest and expertise in stroke and rehabilitation), and education (education and training programmes for staff, patients, and carers). These characteristics were held in common within most stroke unit settings and were usually absent from the conventional care setting. The observation that stroke unit care was usually provided in a geographically discrete ward may reflect difficulties in developing coordinated care within a mobile stroke team.[32]

However, several methodological problems exist with this approach to analysing stroke unit services. Firstly, the information was obtained from the trialists who ran the stroke units and we were not able to obtain information from all staff who provided the conven-

tional care. Therefore our findings could be biased by the expectations of the trialists as to which stroke unit features may or may not be effective. Secondly, this was largely a retrospective analysis and in some cases specific questions could not be answered by the trialist or were not explicitly stated in the original published reports. The information provided here may reflect a mixture of both the recollection of factual details and the recall of features which trialists believed were effective. At best, it represents a strictly factual account of service characteristics, while at the worst, it represents a consensus view from the stroke unit trialists as to which features of stroke unit care were important. Although the identification of characteristics which correlate with effective stroke care does not prove that these characteristics dictated that effectiveness, it does provide powerful circumstantial evidence.

Stroke unit outcomes
The primary question of this review was whether organising inpatient stroke care could improve patient outcomes compared with contemporary conventional care. Our results confirm and extend the findings of previous work[5 33]; compared with conventional care organised stroke unit care reduces the odds of death after stroke. This apparent effect, however, is not statistically robust and could be overturned by a relatively small number of unpublished randomised trials.

The observed reduction in the combined adverse outcomes is much more convincing. The reduction in death or the requirement for long term institutional care was statistically robust. While the requirement for long term care is a useful surrogate for disability that is not subject to assessor bias,[34] the absolute rates of institutionalisation will be influenced by national and cultural factors. Our findings indicate that the reduction in the requirement for institutional care was not due to unreasonable hospital discharge policies because the benefits were sustained for up to one year. They also indicate that reduced institutionalisation was a result of fewer patients becoming dependent rather than more dependent patients being discharged home.

The observed reduction in the combined adverse outcome of death or dependency was also statistically robust. However, it is subject to potential observer bias where final assessments were not carried out in a blinded manner. The sensitivity analysis based on those trials which used an unequivocal blinded assessment suggest that such bias has not seriously influenced the results.

Subgroup analysis
The subgroup analysis indicates that the observed benefits of organised stroke unit care are not limited to any particular subgroup of patients or models of stroke unit organisation. The apparent benefits of stroke unit care were seen in both sexes, in patients aged under and over 75 years, and across a range of stroke severities. Combined acute and rehabilitation stroke units, rehabilitation stroke units, and mixed assessment/rehabilitation units all tended to be more effective than conventional care provided in a general medical ward setting. The limited amount of information from direct comparisons of dedicated stroke rehabilitation units with mixed assessment/rehabilitation unit was insufficient to provide conclusive results. Apparent benefits

were seen in units with acute admission policies as well as those with delayed admission policies and in units operating within different departments.

Rational arguments can be made to support individual models of stroke unit care (for example, combined acute/rehabilitation units are likely to cater for a broader group of stroke patients, mixed assessment/rehabilitation units are more flexible in also offering a service to other patient groups). However, our analysis cannot indicate if one model of specialist stroke unit care is more effective than another. The aspects of care which were held in common by all stroke units concerned their provision of prolonged (up to several weeks) periods of rehabilitation and certain practices and procedures (such as the presence of a coordinated multidisciplinary team approach with specialist stroke interests of medical and nursing staff and programmes of ongoing training and education in stroke). All these aspects of stroke unit care are sufficiently fundamental to permit a flexible approach to improving services but are sufficiently specific to allow the audit of such stroke services.

Cost effectiveness

The results reported here indicate that relatively few stroke patients need to be managed in an organised stroke unit to prevent a death, dependency, or institutionalisation. Our calculations of the number of patients needed to treat to prevent one adverse outcome are very approximate. However, they do indicate the potential degree of benefit which might be achieved through improvements in the organisation of stroke patient care. This compares favourably with many routine medical interventions. However, at what cost would this be achieved?

There are insufficient reliable data available to permit a detailed cost effectiveness analysis of stroke unit care, although recent studies from Canada and Europe indicate that the main costs of inpatient stroke care are due to "hotel" and staffing costs.[35][36] Therefore the length of stay in hospital may be a good surrogate measure of costs assuming that staffing levels are relatively constant. Our analysis of length of stay was complicated by varying definitions of inpatient stay with variable periods of follow up and different approaches to reporting results. However, the benefits of organised stroke unit care did not depend on an increased hospital stay and may even reduce it. It seems reasonable to conclude that organised (stroke unit) care is unlikely to be more expensive than conventional care in a general ward setting and may be less expensive.

Implications

Acute stroke patients should be offered early organised multidisciplinary care, ideally provided within a ward dedicated to stroke care, which can offer a substantial period of rehabilitation if required. Access should not be restricted by age, sex, or stroke severity. There are several approaches to providing this care but all stroke units should aim to replicate the main characteristics of those in the randomised trials.

Future trials should focus on examining the potentially important components of care and on direct comparisons of different models of organised stroke unit care. Preplanned collaboration between compara-

---

Key messages

- Previous systematic reviews of organised inpatient (stroke unit) care have been limited by problems of interpretation and characterising stroke unit care

- The important characteristics of stroke unit care within the randomised trials were the provision of coordinated multidisciplinary rehabilitation, staff specialisation in stroke or rehabilitation, and improved education and training

- Patients managed in a stroke unit were more likely to survive, regain independence, and return home than those receiving conventional care

- Apparent benefits were not restricted to any subgroup of stroke patients or model of stroke unit care

- No systematic increase in length of stay was observed

---

ble trials could alleviate some of the problems of retrospective systematic review.[37]

We thank Carl Counsell and Hazel Fraser (Cochrane Collaboration Stroke Group) for invaluable assistance with literature searching and Patricia Kelly for secretarial support.

List of collaborators (in alphabetical order): K Asplund (Umea, Sweden), P Berman (Nottingham), C Blomstrand (Gothenberg, Sweden), M Dennis (Edinburgh), J Douglas (Glasgow), T Erila (Tampere, Finland), M Garraway (Edinburgh), E Hamrin (Linkoping, Sweden), G Hankey (Perth, Australia), M Ilmavirta (Jyvaskyla, Finland), B Indredavik (Trondheim, Norway), L Kalra (Orpington), M Kaste (Helsinki, Finland), P Langhorne (Glasgow), H Rodgers (Newcastle), J Sivenius (Kuopio, Finland), J Slattery (Edinburgh), R Stevens (Dover), A Svensson (Gothenborg, Sweden), C Warlow (Glasgow), B Williams (Glasgow), S Wood-Dauphinee (Montreal, Canada). Important contributions were also made by D Deleo (Perth, Australia), A Drummond (Nottingham), R Fogelholm (Jyvaskvla, Finland), H Palomaki (Helsinki, Finland), T Strand (Umea, Sweden), and L Wilhelmsen (Gothenberg, Sweden).

Conflict of interest: None.

Funding: Chest, Heart and Stroke, Scotland.

1 Ebrahim S. Does rehabilitation work? In: Ebrahim S, ed. *Clinical epidemiology of stroke.* Oxford: Oxford University Press, 1990:116-21.
2 Mulrow CD. Rationale for systematic reviews. *BMJ* 1994;309:597-9.
3 Stroke Unit Trialists' Collaboration. A systematic overview of specialist multidisciplinary team (stroke unit) care for stroke inpatients. *Cochrane Database of Systematic Reviews;* Disk Issue 1, 1995.
4 Wade D. Activities of daily living (ADL) and extended ADL tests. In: Wade D, ed. *Measurement in neurological rehabilitation.* Oxford: Oxford University Press, 1990:175-94.
5 Wade D, Hewer RL. Functional abilities after stroke: measurement, natural history and prognosis. *J Neurol Neurosurg Psychiatry* 1987;50:177-82.
6 Peto R. Why do we need systematic overviews of randomised trials? *Stat Med* 1987;6:233-40.
7 Thompson SG. Why sources of heterogeneity in meta-analysis should be investigated. *BMJ* 1994;309:1351-5.
8 Der Simonian R, Laird N. Meta-analysis in clinical trials. *Controlled Clin Trials* 1986;7:177-88.
9 Bracken MB. Statistical methods for analysis of effects of treatment in overviews of randomised trials. In: Sinclair JC, Bracken MB, eds. *Effective care of the newborn infant.* Oxford: Oxford University Press, 1992:13-8.
10 Peacock PB, Riley CHP, Lampton TD, Raffel SS, Walker JS. Trends in epidemiology. In: Stewart GT, ed. *The Birmingham stroke, epidemiology and rehabilitation study.* Springfield, Illinois: Thomas, 1972:231-345.
11 Stevens RS, Ambler NR, Warren MD. A randomised controlled trial of a stroke rehabilitation ward. *Age Ageing* 1984;13:65-75.
12 Garraway WM, Akhtar AJ, Hockey L, Prescott RJ. Management of acute stroke in elderly: follow up of a controlled trial. *BMJ* 1980;281:827-9.
13 Svensson A , Harmsen P, Wilhelmsen L. Unpublished data.
14 Fagerberg B, Blomstrand C. Do stroke units save lives? *Lancet* 1993;342:992.
15 Kaste M, Palomaki H, Sarna S. Where and how should elderly stroke patients be treated? A randomised trial. *Stroke* 1995;26:249-53.

16 Gordon EE, Kohn KH. Evaluation of rehabilitation methods in the hemiplegic patient. *J Chron Dis* 1966;19:3-16.

17 Sivenius J, Pyorala K, Heinonen OP, Salonen JT, Riekkinen P. The significance of intensity of rehabilitation after stroke—a controlled trial. *Stroke* 1985;16:928-31.

18 Wood-Dauphinee S, Shapiro S, Bass E, Fletcher C, Georges P, Hensby V, *et al.* A randomised trial of team care following stroke. *Stroke* 1984;5:864-72.

19 Feldman DJ, Lee PR, Unterecker J, Lloyd K, Rusk HA, Toole A. A comparison of functionally orientated medical care and formal rehabilitation in the management of patients with hemiplegia due to cerebrovascular disease. *J Chron Dis* 1962;15:297-310.

20 Aitken PD, Rodgers H, French JM, Bates D, James OFW. General medical or geriatric unit care for acute stroke? A controlled trial. *Age Ageing* 1993;22(suppl 2):4-5.

21 Juby LC, Lincoln NB, Berman P. The effect of a stroke rehabilitation unit on functional and psychological outcome. A randomised controlled trial. *Cerebrovasc Dis* 1996;6:106-10.

22 Kalra L, Dale P, Crome P. Improving stroke rehabilitation: a controlled study. *Stroke* 1993;24:1462-7.

23 Kalra L, Eade J. Role of stroke rehabilitation units in managing severe disability after stroke. *Stroke* 1995;26:2031-4.

24 Hankey G, Deleo D, Stewart-Wynne EG. Acute hospital care for stroke patients: a randomised trial. *Cerebrovasc Dis* 1995;5:228.

25 Ilmavirta M, Frey H, Erila T, Fogelholm R. Stroke outcome and outcome of brain infarction. A prospective randomised study comparing the outcome of patients with brain infarction treated in a stroke unit and in an ordinary neurological ward [academic dissertation]. Tampere: University of Tampere Faculty of Medicine, 1994. (Series A, vol 410.)

26 Indredavik B, Bakke R, Solberg R, Rokseth R, Haahein LL, Home I. Benefit of stroke unit: a randomised controlled trial. *Stroke* 1991;22:1026-31.

27 Strand T, Asplund K, Eriksson S, Hagg E, Lithner F, Wester PO. A non-intensive stroke unit reduced functional disability and the need for long-term hospitalisation. *Stroke* 1985;16:29-34.

28 Hamrin E. Early activation after stroke: does it make a difference? *Scand J Rehabil Med* 1982;14:101-9.

29 Antiplatelet Trialists' Collaboration. Collaborative overview of randomised trials of antiplatelet therapy. 1. Prevention of death, myocardial infarction and stroke by prolonged antiplatelet therapy in various categories of patients. *BMJ* 1994;308:81-106.

30 Chalmers TC, Frank CS, Reitman D. Minimizing the three stages of publication bias. *JAMA* 1990;263:1392-5.

31 Stewart LA, Parmar MKB. Meta-analysis of the literature or of individual patient data: is there a difference? *Lancet* 1993;341:418-22.

32 Dennis MS, Langhorne P. So stroke units save lives? Where do we go from here? *BMJ* 1994; 309:1273-7.

33 Langhorne P, Williams BO, Gilchrist W, Howie K. Do stroke units save lives? *Lancet* 1993;342:395-8.

34 Barer D, Gibson P, Ellul J and the GUESS Group. Outcome of hospital care for stroke in 12 centres. *Age Ageing* 1993;22(suppl 3):15.

35 Smurawska LT, Alexandrov MD, Bladin CF, Norris JW. Cost of acute stroke care in Toronto, Canada. *Stroke* 1994;25:1628-31.

36 Bergman L, van der Meulen JHP, Limburg M, Habbema JDF. Costs of medical care after first-ever stroke in the Netherlands. *Stroke* 1995;26:1830-6.

37 Gladman J, Barer D, Langhorne P. Sepecialist rehabilitation after stroke. *BMJ* 1996;312:1623-4.

(Accepted 24 January 1997)

Citation:

Are the results of this systematic review of therapy valid?

Is it a systematic review of randomised trials of the treatment you're interested in?

Does it include a methods section that describes:

- finding and including all the relevant trials?

- assessing their individual validity?

Were the results consistent from study to study?

Are the valid results of this systematic review important?

Translating odds ratios to NNTs. The numbers in the body of the table are the NNTs for the corresponding odds ratios at that particular patient's expected event rate (PEER).

		Odds ratios (OR)								
		0.9	0.85	0.8	0.75	0.7	0.65	0.6	0.55	0.5
	.05	209[1]	139	104	83	69	59	52	46	41[2]
	.10	110	73	54	43	36	31	27	24	21
Control	.20	61	40	30	24	20	17	14	13	11
Event	.30	46	30	22	18	14	12	10	9	8
Rate	.40	40	26	19	15	12	10	9	8	7
(CER)	.50[3]	38	25	18	14	11	9	8	7	6
	.70	44	28	20	16	13	10	9	7	6
	.90	101[4]	64	46	34	27	22	18	15	12[5]

[1] The relative risk reduction (RRR) here is 10%

[2] The RRR here is 49%

[3] For any OR, NNT is lowest when PEER = .50

[4] The RRR here is 1%

[5] The RRR here is 9%

Can you apply this valid, important evidence from a systematic review in caring for your patient?

Do these results apply to your patient?

Is your patient so different from those in the
systematic review that its results can't help you?

How great would the potential benefit of therapy actually be for your individual patient?

Method I: In the table on page 1, find the
intersection of the closest odds ratio from the
systematic review and the CER that is closest to your
patient's expected event rate if they received the
control treatment (PEER):

Method II: To calculate the NNT for any OR and PEER:

$$NNT = \frac{1 - \{PEER \times (1 - OR)\}}{(1 - PEER) \times PEER \times (1 - OR)}$$

Are your patient's values and preferences satisfied by the regimen and its consequences?

Do you and your patient have a clear assessment
of their values and preferences?

Are they met by this regimen and its consequences?

Should you believe apparent qualitative differences in the efficacy of therapy in some subgroups of patients? Only if you can say 'yes' to all of the following:

Do they really make biologic and clinical sense?

Is the qualitative difference both clinically (beneficial
for some but useless or harmful for others) and
statistically significant?

Was this difference hypothesised before the study
began (rather than the product of dredging the
data), and has it been confirmed in other,
independent studies?

Was this one of just a few subgroup analyses carried
out in this study?

Additional notes

Citation: Stroke Unit Trialists' Collaboration (1997) Collaborative systematic review of the randomised trials of organised inpatient (stroke unit) care after stroke. *BMJ.* **314: 1151–9.**

Are the results of this systematic review (systematic review) of therapy valid?

Is it a systematic review of randomised trials of the treatment you're interested in?	**Yes.**

Does it include a methods section that describes:

• finding and including all the relevant trials?	**Yes.**
• assessing their individual validity?	**No, but does include characteristics of individual trials.**

Were the results consistent from study to study?	**Consistent results when death is the outcome, when death or dependency is the outcome, some heterogeneity but this was explored and seems to reflect the nature of the control group, i.e. less heterogeneity when the stroke unit group was compared to a general medical unit. There was significant heterogeneity in length of stay.**

Are the valid results of this systematic review important?

Translating odds ratios to NNTs. The numbers in the body of the table are the NNTs for the corresponding odds ratios at that particular patient's expected event rate (PEER).

		Odds ratios (OR)								
		0.9	0.85	0.8	0.75	0.7	0.65	0.6	0.55	0.5
	.05	209[1]	139	104	83	69	59	52	46	41[2]
	.10	110	73	54	43	36	31	27	24	21
Control	.20	61	40	30	24	20	17	14	13	11
Event	.30	46	30	22	18	14	12	10	9	8
Rate	.40	40	26	19	15	12	10	9	8	7
(CER)	.50[3]	38	25	18	14	11	9	8	7	6
	.70	44	28	20	16	13	10	9	7	6
	.90	101[4]	64	46	34	27	22	18	15	12[5]

[1] The relative risk reduction (RRR) here is 10%

[2] The RRR here is 49%

[3] For any OR, NNT is lowest when PEER = .50

[4] The RRR here is 1%

[5] The RRR here is 9%

Can you apply this valid, important evidence from a systematic review in caring for your patient?

Do these results apply to your patient?

Is your patient so different from those in the systematic review that its results can't help you?	**No.**

How great would the potential benefit of therapy actually be for your individual patient?

Method I: In the table on page 1, find the intersection of the closest odds ratio from the overview and the CER that is closest to your patient's expected event rate if they received the control treatment (PEER):	**EER (0.679) and CER (0.611) provided in** *Best Evidence*. **For death and dependency the NNT is 15 (12 to 41).**

Method II: To calculate the NNT for any OR and PEER:

$$NNT = \frac{1 - \{PEER \times (1 - OR)\}}{(1 - PEER) \times PEER \times (1 - OR)}$$

Are your patient's values and preferences satisfied by the regimen and its consequences?

Do you and your patient have a clear assessment of their values and preferences?	**Needs to be assessed in each patient.**
Are they met by this regimen and its consequences?	**Needs to be assessed in each patient.**

Should you believe apparent qualitative differences in the efficacy of therapy in some subgroups of patients? Only if you can say 'yes' to all of the following:

Do they really make biologic and clinical sense?	**Yes.**
Is the qualitative difference both clinically (beneficial for some but useless or harmful for others) and statistically significant?	**Yes.**
Was this difference hypothesised before the study began (rather than the product of dredging the data), and has it been confirmed in other, independent studies?	**Yes.**
Was this one of just a few subgroup analyses carried out in this study?	**Yes.**

Additional notes

Clinical Bottom Line

Stroke units decrease death and dependency, and death and institutionalisation.

Citation

Stroke Unit Trialists' Collaboration (1997) Collaborative systematic review of the randomised trials of organised inpatient (stroke unit) care after stroke. *BMJ*. **314:** 1151–9.

Three-part Question

In a patient with a stroke, does admission to a stroke unit decrease the risk of death and dependency?

Search Terms

'stroke unit' and 'death' in *Best Evidence*.

The Study

Systematic review of RCTs that studied dedicated stroke units, mixed assessment and rehab units or general medical wards with outcomes of death, dependency or institutionalisation.

The Evidence

19 trials including 3249 patients.

Outcomes*	CER (weighted)	EER (weighted)	RRR (95% CI)	ARR (weighted)	NNT (95% CI)
Death and dependency	.679	.611	9% (16 to 39)	.068	15 (12 to 41)
Death and institutionalisation	.475	.377	18% (6 to 28)	.098	11 (7 to 32)

*Dependency defined as the need for physical assistance with transfers, mobility, feeding, dressing or toileting. Institutionalisation included nursing home placement, residential care placement or hospitalisation at the end of the rehab period.

Comments

1 Mortality rate 21% in the stroke unit and 25% in the general medicine group.

2 Heterogeneity in death or dependency amongst the trials but seems to reflect the nature of the control group.

3 Advantages as great in older patients as in younger patients and in those who have had severe stroke as in those who have had milder strokes.

4 Little difference in staff numbers or mix or in intensity of rehab provided in organised vs conventional care settings but tendency for assessment and treatment to begin earlier in organised settings.

5 Most significant difference were the degree of specialised medical and nursing interest in stroke, staff training and involvement of family and caregivers in the rehab process.

STROKE –
STROKE UNITS
DECREASE DEATH,
DEPENDENCY AND
INSTITUTIONAL-
ISATION

Appraised by Sharon Straus: 1998.
Expiry date: 2000.

PART A

Presentations
(comfortably 3 per hour)

1   In groups of 10 or less, participants will present their critical appraisals they have carried out on clinical topics of their choice.

2   Reports will state the three-part clinical question, summarise the search in one sentence, critically appraise the best article found, and discuss how the appraisal was integrated with clinical expertise and applied on that (or a similar, subsequent) patient.

3   A total of 15 minutes will be allotted for each presentation: 10 minutes for presentation and 5 minutes for group discussion.

PART B

Searching for evidence on the WWW

We will show you how to access the web and introduce you to the web page for the Centre for Evidence-Based Medicine in Oxford (http://cebm.jr2.ox.ac.uk/), where there are data banks of clinically useful measures on the precision and accuracy of clinical exam and lab test results (SpPins, SnNouts, sensitivities, specificities, likelihood ratios), the power of prognostic factors and therapy (NNTs, RRRs and the like), plus the CATMaker and links to several other centres and sources of evidence.

NOTES ON THE INTERNET

The Internet: why bother?

- Networking with colleagues.
- Getting hold of useful documents for free.
- Publishing useful information for free.
- Bypassing traditional publishers and online vendors.

EBM on the Internet

- e-mail discussion list (run by Mailbase):
  evidence-based-health@mailbase.ac.uk

To join send an e-mail to **mailbase@mailbase.ac.uk** with an empty subject field and the following as the only text of the message itself: **join evidence-based-health Joe Bloggs**

To get list of mailbase discussion lists, send this command in the same way to the same address: **find lists medical**

To get a mailbase user guide, send the command: **send mailbase user-guide**

- The EBM Toolbox (the CEBM World-Wide Web site)
  http://cebm.jr2.ox.ac.uk/

See links to other sites (especially SCHARR) in Other Resources. It also has:

- a glossary of EBHC terms and research methodologies
- how to focus a clinical question
- educational prescriptions
- hints on how to optimise MEDLINE searches
- detailed definitions and examples of NNTs, SpPins and SnNouts, likelihood ratios, pre-test probabilities, prognostic indicators
- scenarios used in the teaching packs at our workshops
- worksheets for critical appraisal

Searching for stuff on the Web

- Use other people's links to good sites. An excellent place to start for this is the Netting the Evidence and SCHARR Project at Sheffield:
  http://www.shef.ac.uk/~scharr/ir/netting.html
- To find your own good sites, use the search engines, such as:

Altavista:	**www.altavista.com**
Excite:	**www.excite.com**
Lycos:	**www.lycos.com**
Yahoo!:	**www.yahoo.com**

There is a good site with links to all the best internet search engines at: **http://alt.venus.co.uk/weed/search/welcome.htm**

- The browser's **Find** button can help to scan large pages
- Use **Bookmarks** to record good sites
- You can search MEDLINE on the Internet at various sites, including PubMed: **http://www3.ncbi.nlm.nih.gov/PubMed/**

TCP/IP (Transmission Control Protocol / Internet Protocol): the lingua franca, a common language of protocols which allows different computers to exchange information.

- It is a loose association of networks of computers which has generated a massive publishing and communications arena.

- Every computer on the Internet (host) has its own unique IP address which defines where it is and enables other computers to send and forward messages to it. There is no central server for the Internet, so it is both robust (nearly impossible to destroy) and chaotic (nearly impossible to control).

- Typically, you will use your computer to log in to a host which has an Internet connection and which has an account for your use. If you are lucky, your machine will be a host in itself, which means others can log in to your machine and use it (for example, see Telnet).

- You will use the Internet from a particular domain (locality) which will have local management of services.

- the set of five services which are supported by the Internet protocols are:

E-mail (SMTP)	Text messages sent to a person: **user@host.domain**	User decides when to read, one to many with mailing lists, e.g. mailbase.	Not 100% reliable; Internet e-mail not universal in NHS; addresses can be obscure.
USENET News Groups (NNTP)	USENET servers contain textual discussion lists where users add their comments to a discussion.	Thousands of topics to choose from; can be a good source of advice.	Difficult to find relevant group; can be a source of abuse!
Telnet	Allows you to connect to a host computer across the Internet and use it as if you were sitting in front of it.	Allows you to use the resources of the host computer.	Usually just text-based commands, i.e. no Windows; you need an account with the host to be able to do this.
File transfer protocol (FTP)	You can log on to a host, browse its directories and exchange files efficiently (including programs).	You don't need authorisation (anonymous FTP means you type 'Guest' as a login name and your e-mail address as password).	Can be very difficult to browse effectively (you have to know where to look and download to see what you are getting).
WWW (http)	Use a browser program to read multimedia documents (and programs) stored on any Internet host running the http program.	Instant publishing. Login, addressing and downloading with one click of the mouse. Can be searched and marked.	Imagine the Bodleian with all the books shuffled and dumped on the floor.

Usually, different services will be managed locally by a specific host (a server) which may or may not be the same machine.

Reference
Krol E (1994) The Whole Internet: users' guide and catalogue. O'Reilly.

PART A | Presentations

The other half of the participants will present their patients, questions, critically appraised topics, and clinical conclusions.

PART B | Feedback and celebration

The final portion of the session (and course!) can be spent evaluating the course. The first of the attached forms (**Evaluation of 'practising EBM'**) permits written feedback about this course, and a discussion will be held on the general issues within it.

The second form (**'Am I practising EBM?'**) is a checklist that you may want to apply to your own performance in order to determine whether you are beginning to apply the self-directed, problem-based learning and EBM skills in your own practice and in your clinical teaching.

Special attention will be given to discussing and deciding what to do with what has been learned, and how to continue to improve and use this set of clinical, EBM and self-directed learning skills.

EVALUATION OF 'PRACTISING EBM'

Please rate the items using the following scale from 1 to 5 where:

1 – awful   3 – adequate   5 – excellent

1   *How well were your objectives met in this course?*

a   Learning how to ask answerable clinical questions related to pts you care for on the clinical service

1	2	3	4	5

b   Learning how to search for the best evidence

1	2	3	4	5

c   Learning how to critically appraise the medical literature

1	2	3	4	5

d   Learning how to integrate this literature with your clinical expertise and to apply the results in your clinical practice

1	2	3	4	5

e   Learning how to evaluate your performance

1	2	3	4	5

2   *Therapy Session*

a	Relevance of the session	1	2	3	4	5
b	Appropriateness of the article	1	2	3	4	5
c	Organisation of the session	1	2	3	4	5
d	Teaching during the session	1	2	3	4	5

3   *Diagnosis Session*

a	Relevance of the session	1	2	3	4	5
b	Appropriateness of the article	1	2	3	4	5
c	Organisation of the session	1	2	3	4	5
d	Teaching during the session	1	2	3	4	5

3   *Prognosis Session*

a	Relevance of the session	1	2	3	4	5
b	Appropriateness of the article	1	2	3	4	5
c	Organisation of the session	1	2	3	4	5
d	Teaching during the session	1	2	3	4	5

4   *Systematic Review Session*

a	Relevance of the session	1	2	3	4	5
b	Appropriateness of the article	1	2	3	4	5
c	Organisation of the session	1	2	3	4	5
d	Teaching during the session	1	2	3	4	5

5 *Harm Session*

   a Relevance of the session   1   2   3   4   5

   b Appropriateness of the article   1   2   3   4   5

   c Organisation of the session   1   2   3   4   5

   d Teaching during the session   1   2   3   4   5

6 *Final Presentation Sessions*

   a Relevance of the presentations   1   2   3   4   5

   b Quality of the presentations   1   2   3   4   5

   c Quality of the discussions   1   2   3   4   5

   d Organisation of the session   1   2   3   4   5

7 *How well do you think this course will help you prepare for your Membership Exams?*

                              1   2   3   4   5

8 *Overall rating of the course*

                              1   2   3   4   5

9 *What was the best thing about this course*
   (that should be preserved and expanded in future courses)?

10 *What was the worst thing about this course*
   (that should be removed from future courses of this sort)?

11 *Other comments and suggestions:*

Many thanks

AM I PRACTISING EBM?

A self-evaluation in asking answerable questions.

a Are you asking any questions at all?

b Are you:
- using the guides to asking 3-part questions?
- using educational prescriptions
- asking your colleagues: 'What's your evidence for that?'

c Is your success rate of asking answerable questions rising?

d How do your questions compare with those of respected colleagues?

A self-evaluation in finding the best external evidence.

a Are you searching at all?

b Do you know the best sources of current evidence for your clinical discipline?

c Have you achieved immediate access to searching hardware, software and the best evidence for your clinical discipline?

d Are you finding useful external evidence from a widening array of sources?

e Are you becoming more efficient in your searching?

f Are you using MeSH headings, thesaurus, limiters, and intelligent free text when searching MEDLINE?

g How do your searches compare with those of research librarians or other respected colleagues who have a passion for providing best current patient care?

A self-evaluation in critically appraising the evidence for its validity and potential usefulness.

a Are you critically appraising external evidence at all?

b Are the critical appraisal guides becoming easier to apply?

c Are you becoming more accurate and efficient in applying some of the critical appraisal measures (such as likelihood ratios, NNTs and the like)?

d Are you creating any CATs?

e Are you using the CATMaker?

f Have you shared any of the CATs you've made with your colleagues or other learners?

A self-evaluation in integrating the critical appraisal with your clinical expertise and applying the result in your clinical practice.

a Are you integrating your critical appraisals into your practice at all?

b Are you becoming more accurate and efficient in adjusting some of the critical appraisal measures to fit your individual patients (pre-test probabilities, NNT/f, etc.)?

c Can you explain (and resolve) disagreements about management decisions in terms of this integration?

d Have you conducted any clinical decision analyses?

e Have you carried out any audits of your diagnostic, therapeutic, or other EBM performance?

A self-evaluation in teaching EBM.

a   When did you last issue an educational prescription?

b   Are you helping your trainees learn how to ask answerable (3-part) questions?

c   Are you teaching and modelling searching skills (or making sure that your trainees learn them)?

d   Are you teaching and modelling critical appraisal skills?

e   Are you teaching and modelling the generation of CATs?

f   Are you teaching and modelling the integration of best evidence with individual clinical expertise?

g   Are you developing new ways of evaluating the effectiveness of your teaching?[1]

h   Are you developing new EBM educational materials?[2]

A self-evaluation of your own continuing professional development.

a   Are you a member of an EBM-style journal club?

b   Have you participated in or tutored at one of the workshops on how to practice or teach EBM?

c   Have you joined the evidence-based-health e-mail discussion group?

d   Have you established links with other practitioners or teachers of EBM?

[1] If so, please share them with the developers of this course!

[2] If so, please add them to the bank of EBM educational resources that the Oxford Centre for Evidence-based Medicine shares with other educators around the world.

Glossary of terms you are likely to encounter in your clinical reading

This glossary is intended to provide guidance as to the meanings of terms you will come across frequently in clinical articles, especially when they appear in EBM journals.

Absolute risk reduction (ARR) – see **Treatment effects**

Case-control study – a study which involves identifying patients who have the outcome of interest (cases) and control patients without the same outcome, and looking back to see if they had the exposure of interest (see also **Review of study designs**).

Case-series – a report on a series of patients with an outcome of interest. No control group is involved.

Clinical practice guideline – is a systematically developed statement designed to assist practitioner and patient decisions about appropriate health care for specific clinical circumstances.

Cohort study – involves identification of two groups (cohorts) of patients, one which did receive the exposure of interest, and one which did not, and following these cohorts forward for the outcome of interest (see also **Review of study designs**).

Confidence interval (CI) – the range within which we would expect the true value of a statistical measure to lie. The CI is usually accompanied by a percentage value which shows the level of confidence that the true value lies within this range. For example, for an NNT of 10 with a 95% CI of 5 to 15, we would have 95% confidence that the true NNT value was between 5 and 15.

Control event rate (CER) – see **Treatment effects**.

Cost-benefit analysis – assesses whether the cost of an intervention is worth the benefit by measuring both in the same units; monetary units are usually used.

Cost-effectiveness analysis – measures the net cost of providing a service as well as the outcomes obtained. Outcomes are reported in a single unit of measurement.

Cost-minimisation analysis – if health effects are known to be equal, only costs are analysed and the least costly alternative is shown.

Cost-utility analysis – converts effects into personal preferences (or utilities) and describes how much it costs for some additional quality gain (e.g. cost per additional quality-adjusted life-year, or QALY).

Crossover study design – the administration of two or more experimental therapies one after the other in a specified or random order to the same group of patients (see also **Review of study designs**).

Cross-sectional study – the observation of a defined population at a single point in time or time interval. Exposure and outcome are determined simultaneously (*see also* **Review of study designs**).

Decision analysis – is the application of explicit, quantitative methods that quantify prognoses, treatment effects, and patient values in order to analyse a decision under conditions of uncertainty.

Ecological survey – a survey based on aggregated data for some population as it exists at some point or points in time; to investigate the relationship of an exposure to a known or presumed risk factor for a specified outcome.

Event rate – the proportion of patients in a group in whom the event is observed. Thus, if out of 100 patients, the event is observed in 27, the event rate is 0.27. Control event rate (CER) and experimental event rate (EER) are used to refer to this in control and experimental groups of patients respectively. The patient expected event rate (PEER) refers to the rate of events we'd expect in a patient who received no treatment or conventional treatment – *see* **Treatment effects**.

Evidence-based health care – extends the application of the principles of evidence-based medicine (*see* below) to all professions associated with health care, including purchasing and management.

Evidence-based medicine – the conscientious, explicit and judicious use of current best evidence in making decisions about the care of individual patients. The practice of evidence-based medicine means integrating individual clinical expertise with the best available external clinical evidence from systematic research. *See also* Sackett *et al.* (1996) EBM: What it is and what it isn't. *BMJ* **312:** 71–2.

Experimental event rate (EER) – *see* **Treatment effects**.

Inception cohort – a group of patients assembled near the onset of the target disorder.

Incidence – the proportion of new cases of the target disorder in the population at risk during a specified time interval.

Intention to treat analysis – a method of analysis for randomised trials in which all patients randomly assigned to one of the treatments are analysed together, regardless of whether or not they completed or received that treatment.

Likelihood ratio (LR) – the likelihood that a given test result would be expected in a patient with the target disorder compared to the likelihood that that same result would be expected in a patient without the target disorder.

Calculation of sensitivity/specificity/LR:

	DISEASE POSITIVE	**DISEASE NEGATIVE**
TEST POSITIVE	a	b
TEST NEGATIVE	c	d

Sensitivity = a/(a+c)

$$LR+ = \frac{sensitivity}{1-specificity} = \frac{a/(a+c)}{b/(b+d)}$$

Specificity = d/(b+d)

$$LR- = \frac{(1-sensitivity)}{specificity} = \frac{c/(a+c)}{d/(b+d)}$$

Positive predictive value = a/(a+b)   Negative predictive value = d/(c+d)

Meta-analysis – is a systematic review that uses quantitative methods to summarise the results.

N-of-1 trials – in such trials, the patient undergoes pairs of treatment periods organised so that one period involves the use of the experimental treatment and one period involves the use of an alternate or placebo therapy. The patients and physician are blinded, if possible, and outcomes are monitored. Treatment periods are replicated until the clinician and patient are convinced that the treatments are definitely different or definitely not different.

Negative predictive value – proportion of people with a negative test who are free of the target disorder (*see also* **Likelihood ratio**).

Number needed to treat (NNT) – is the inverse of the absolute risk reduction and is the number of patients that need to be treated to prevent one bad outcome – *see* **Treatment effects**.

Odds – a ratio of non-events to events. If the event rate for a disease is 0.1 (10%), its non-event rate is 0.9 and therefore its odds are 9:1. Note that this is not the same expression as the inverse of event rate.

Odds ratio (OR) – is the odds of having the target disorder in the experimental group relative to the odds in favour of having the target disorder in the control group (in prospective case-control studies, overviews) or the odds in favour of being exposed in subjects with the target disorder divided by the odds in favour of being exposed in control subjects (without the target disorder).

Calculations of OR/RR for use of trimethoprim-sulfamethoxazole prophylaxis in cirrhosis:

	Adverse event occurs (infectious complication)	Adverse event does not occur (no infectious complication)	Totals
Exposed to treatment (experimental)	1 a	29 b	30 a+b
Not exposed to treatment (control)	c 9	d 21	c+d 30
Totals	a+c 10	b+d 50	a+b+c+d 60

CER = c/(c+d) = 0.30
EER = a/(a+b) = 0.033
Control Event Odds = c/d = 0.43
Experimental Event Odds = a/b = 0.034
Relative Risk = EER/CER = 0.11
Relative Odds = Odds Ratio = (a/b)/(c/d) = ad/bc = 0.08

Patient expected event rate – see **Treatment effects**.

Overview – see **Systematic review**.

Positive predictive value – proportion of people with a positive test who have the target disorder (see also **Likelihood ratio**).

Post-test odds – the odds that the patient has the target disorder after the test has been carried out (pre-test odds and likelihood ratio).

Post-test probability – the proportion of patients with that particular test result who have the target disorder.

Pre-test odds – the odds that the patient has the target disorder before the test has been carried out (pre-test probability/1 – pre-test probability).

Pre-test probability/prevalence – the proportion of people with the target disorder in the population at risk at a specific time or time interval.

Randomised controlled clinical trial (RCT) – a group of patients is randomised into an experimental group and a control group. These groups are followed up for the variables / outcomes of interest (see also **Review of study designs**).

Relative risk reduction (RRR) – see **Treatment effects**.

Risk ratio (RR) – is the ratio of risk in the treated group (EER) to the risk in the control group (CER) – used in randomised trials and cohort studies:

$$RR = ERR/CER$$

Sensitivity – proportion of people with the target disorder who have a positive test. It is used to assist in assessing and selecting a diagnostic test/sign/symptom (*see also **Likelihood ratio***).

SnNout – when a sign/test/symptom has a high **S**ensitivity, a **N**egative result rules **out** the diagnosis, e.g. the sensitivity of a history of ankle swelling for diagnosing ascites is 93%, therefore if a person does not have a history of ankle swelling, it is highly unlikely that the person has ascites.

Specificity – proportion of people without the target disorder who have a negative test. It is used to assist in assessing and selecting a diagnostic test/sign/symptom (*see also **Likelihood ratio***).

SpPin – when a sign/test/symptom has a high **S**pecificity, a **P**ositive result rules **in** the diagnosis, e.g. the specificity of a fluid wave for diagnosing ascites is 92%, therefore if a person does have a fluid wave, it rules in the diagnosis of ascites

Systematic review – a summary of the medical literature that uses explicit methods to perform a thorough literature search and critical appraisal of individual studies, and that uses appropriate statistical techniques to combine these valid studies.

Treatment effects

The E-B journals have achieved consensus on some terms they use to describe both the good and the bad effects of therapy. They will join the terms already in current use (RRR, ARR, NNT), and both sets are described here and summarised in the Glossary that appears inside the back cover of *Evidence-based Medicine*. We will bring them to life with a synthesis of three randomised trials in diabetes which individually showed that several years of intensive insulin therapy reduced the proportion of patients with worsening retinopathy to 13% from 38%, raised the proportion of patients with satisfactory haemoglobin A1c levels to 60% from about 30%, and increased the proportion of patients with at least one episode of symptomatic hypoglycaemia to 47% from 23%. Note that in each case the first number constitutes the 'experimental event rate' or EER and the second number the 'control event rate' or CER. We will use the following terms and calculations to describe these effects of treatment:

When the experimental treatment reduces the probability of a bad outcome (worsening diabetic retinopathy).

RRR (Relative risk reduction): the proportional reduction in rates of bad outcomes between experimental and control participants in a trial, calculated as |EER – CER|/CER, and accompanied by a 95% confidence interval (CI). In the case of worsening diabetic retinopathy, |EE – CER|/CER = |13% – 38%|/38% = 66%.

ARR (Absolute risk reduction): the absolute arithmetic difference in rates of bad outcomes between experimental and control participants in a trial, calculated as IEER − CERI, and accompanied by a 95% CI. In this case, IEER − CERI = I13% − 38%I = 25%.

NNT (Number needed to treat): the number of patients who need to be treated to achieve 1 additional favourable outcome, calculated as 1/ARR and accompanied by a 95% CI. In this case, 1/ARR = 1/25% = 4.

Calculations for the occurrence of diabetic retinopathy in IDDMs:

Occurrence of diabetic neuropathy at 5 yr among insulin-dependent diabetics in the DCCT trial		Relative risk reduction (RRR)	Absolute risk reduction (ARR)	Number needed to treat (NNT)
Usual insulin regimen CER	Intensive insulin regimen EER	$\dfrac{\text{IEER} - \text{CERI}}{\text{CER}}$	IEER − CERI	1/ARR
13%	38%	I13% − 38%I / 38% = 66%	I13% − 38%I = 25%	1/25% = 4 pts, for 6 years, with intensive insulin Rx

When the experimental treatment increases the probability of a good outcome (satisfactory haemoglobin A1c levels).

RBI (Relative benefit increase): the proportional increase in rates of good outcomes between experimental and control patients in a trial, calculated as IEER-CERI/CER, and accompanied by a 95% confidence interval (CI). In the case of satisfactory haemoglobin A1c levels, IEER − CERI/CER = I60% − 30%I/30% = 100%.

ABI (Absolute benefit increase): the absolute arithmetic difference in rates of good outcomes between experimental and control patients in a trial, calculated as IEER − CERI, and accompanied by a 95% CI. In the case of satisfactory haemoglobin A1c levels, IEER − CERI = I60% − 30%I = 30%.

NNT (Number needed to treat): The number of patients who need to be treated to achieve one additional good outcome, calculated as 1/ARR and accompanied by a 95% CI. In this case, 1/ARR = 1/30% = 3.

When the experimental treatment increase the probability of a bad outcome (episodes of hypoglycaemia).

RRI (Relative risk increase): the proportional increase in rates of bad outcomes between experimental and control patients in a trial, calculated as IEER − CERI/CER, and accompanied by a 95% CI. In the case of hypoglycaemic episodes, IEER − CERI/CER = I57% − 23%I/57% = 34%/57% = 60%. (RRI is also used in assessing the impact of 'risk factors' for disease.)

ARI (Absolute risk increase): the absolute arithmetic difference in rates of bad outcomes between experimental and control patients in a trial, calculated as IEER – CERI, and accompanied by a 95% CI. In the case of hypoglycaemic episodes, IEER – CERI = I57% – 23%I = 34%. (ARI is also used in assessing the impact of 'risk factors' for disease.)

NNH (Number needed to harm): the number of patients who, if they received the experimental treatment, would lead to one additional patient being harmed, compared with patients who received the control treatment, calculated as 1/ARR and accompanied by a 95% CI. In this case, 1/ARR = 1/34% = 3.

		Adverse Outcome		Totals
		Present (case)	**Absent (control)**	
Exposed to the Treatment	Yes (cohort)	a	b	a+b
	No (cohort)	c	d	c+d
	Totals	a+c	b+d	a+b+c+d

In a randomised trial or cohort study:
Relative risk = RR = $[a/(a+b)]/[c/(c+d)]$

In a case-control study:
Odds ratio (or Relative odds) = OR = ad/bc

Randomized controlled trial: start with a+b+c+d and randomise to (a+b) and (c+d)

Advantages

1 Assignment to treatment can be kept concealed.

2 Confounders equally distributed.

3 Blinding more likely.

4 Randomisation facilitates statistical analysis.

Disadvantages

1 Expensive – time and money.

2 Volunteer bias.

3 Ethically problematic at times.

Crossover design

Advantages

1 Subjects serve as own controls and error variance is reduced thus reducing sample size needed.

2 All subjects receive treatment (at least some of the time).

3 Statistical tests assuming randomisation can be used.

4 Blinding can be maintained.

Disadvantages

1 All subjects receive placebo or alternative treatment at some point.

2 Washout period lengthy or unknown.

3 Cannot be used for treatments with permanent effects.

Cohort study: selects (a+b) and (c+d)

Advantages

1 Ethically safe.

2 Subjects can be matched.

3 Can establish timing and directionality of events.

4 Eligibility criteria and outcome assessments can be standardised.

5 Administratively easier and cheaper than RCT.

Disadvantages

1 Controls may be difficult to identify.

2 Exposure may be linked to a hidden confounder.

3 Blinding difficult.

4 Still expensive.

5 Randomisation not present.

6 For rare disease, large sample sizes or long follow-up necessary.

Cross-sectional (analytic) survey: selecting a+b+c+d

Advantages

1 Cheap and simple.

2 Safe ethically.

Disadvantages

1 Establishes association at most, not causality.

2 Recall bias susceptibility.

3 Confounders may be unequally distributed.

4 Neyman bias.

5 Group sizes may be unequal.

Case-control study: selecting (a+c) and (b+d)

Advantages

1 Quick and cheap.

2 Only feasible method for very rare disorders or those with long lag between exposure and outcome.

3 Fewer subjects needed than cross-sectional studies.

Disadvantages

1 Reliance on recall or records to determine exposure status.

2 Confounders.

3 Selection of control groups difficult.

4 Potential bias – recall, selection.

Section 3a1

Is this evidence about a diagnostic test valid?

Having found a possibly useful article about a diagnostic test, how can you quickly critically appraise it for its proximity to the truth? This can be done by asking some simple questions; often you'll find their answers in the article's abstract. Table 3a1.1 lists these questions for individual reports, but you can also apply them to the interpretation of a systematic review (overview) of several different studies of the same diagnostic test for the same target disorder.*

The first guide is: 'Was there an independent, blind comparison with a reference ("gold") standard of diagnosis?' This is quite a mouthful, but it simply means that two criteria should have been met. The patients in the study should have undergone *both* the diagnostic test in question (say, an item of the history or physical examination, a blood test, etc.) *and* the reference (or 'gold') standard (an autopsy or biopsy or other confirmatory 'proof' that they do or don't have the target disorder); and the results of one shouldn't be known to those who are applying and interpreting the other (for example, the pathologist interpreting the biopsy that comprises the reference standard for the target disorder should be 'blind' to the result of the blood test that comprises the diagnostic test under study). In this way, investigators avoid the conscious and unconscious bias that otherwise might cause the reference standard to be 'overinterpreted' when the diagnostic test is positive and 'underinterpreted' when it is negative. Sometimes investigators have a difficult time coming up with clearcut

---

* As we'll stress throughout this book, systematic reviews will give you the most valid and useful external evidence on just about any clinical question you can pose. They are still pretty rare for diagnostic tests and for this reason we'll describe them in their usual, therapeutic habitat, in Section 3a3. When using Table 3a3.2 to consider diagnostic tests, simply substitute 'diagnostic test' for 'treatment' as you read.

Table 3a1.1 Are the results of this diagnostic study valid?

1. Was there an independent, blind comparison with a reference ('gold') standard of diagnosis?
2. Was the diagnostic test evaluated in an appropriate spectrum of patients (like those in whom it would be used in practice)?
3. Was the reference standard applied regardless of the diagnostic test result?

reference standards (e.g. for psychiatric disorders) and you'll want to give careful consideration to their arguments justifying the selection of their reference standard.

One way or another, the report will wind up calling some results 'normal' and others 'abnormal' and we'll show you how to interpret these in Section 3b1. For now, you might simply want to recognize that there are six definitions of 'normal' in common use (we've listed them in Table 3a1.2). We will make use of definition 5 ('diagnostic' normal) and believe that half of the definitions are not useful. The first two (the Gaussian and percentile definitions) are derived from the study test results alone, with no reference standard, and simply define the 'normal range' for the diagnostic test result on the basis of statistical properties (standard deviations or percentiles). Thus they are properties of the test in isolation from any objective reality. These don't make any sense to us, for they imply that all 'abnormalities' occur at the same frequency. They both suggest that if we can perform enough diagnostic tests on a patient we are bound to find something 'abnormal' and lead to all sorts of inappropriate further testing. The third definition of 'normal' (culturally desirable) represents a cultural value judgment. It is seen in fashion advertisements and at the fringes of the 'lifestyle' movement where medicine becomes confused with morality. The fourth (risk factor) definition has the drawback that it 'labels' or stigmatizes some patients and is clinically useful only if we can do something positive to lower their risk. The fifth (diagnostic) definition is the one that we will focus on here and we will show you how to generate and interpret diagnostic normality in Section 3b1. The final (therapeutic) definition is in part an outgrowth of the

Table 3a1.2 Six definitions of normal

1. Gaussian: the mean +/- 2 standard deviations. Assumes a normal distribution and means that all 'abnormalities' have the same frequency.
2. Percentile: within the range, say, of 5–95%. Has the same basic defect as the Gaussian definition.
3. Culturally desirable: preferred by society. Confuses the role of medicine.
4. Risk factor: carrying no additional risk of disease. Labels the outliers, who may not be helped.
5. Diagnostic: range of results beyond which target disorders become highly probable – the focus of this discussion.
6. Therapeutic: range of results beyond which treatment does more good than harm. Means you have to keep up with advances in therapy!

fourth (risk factor) definition and has the great clinical advantage that it changes with our knowledge of efficacy. Thus, the definition of normal blood pressure has changed radically over the past few decades as we have learned that treatment of progressively lower blood pressure levels does more good than harm.

Returning to the second question in Table 3a1.1, you will want the diagnostic test to have been evaluated in an appropriate spectrum of patients, similar to the practice population in which the test might be used. Among patients with late or severe disease, when the diagnosis is obvious, often you won't need any diagnostic test, so studies that confine themselves to florid cases are not very informative. The article will be informative if the diagnostic test was applied to patients with mild as well as severe and early as well as late cases of the target disorder and among both treated and untreated individuals. In addition, you would want the diagnostic test to have been applied to patients with different disorders that are commonly confused with the target disorder of interest.

Finally, was the reference standard applied regardless of the diagnostic test result? When patients have a negative diagnostic test result, investigators are tempted to forego applying the reference standard and when the latter is invasive or risky (e.g. angiography) it may be considered inappropriate to do so. For this reason, many investigators now employ a reference standard for a patient *not* having the target disorder in which they *don't* suffer any adverse health outcome during a long follow-up on no definitive treatment (for example, convincing evidence that a patient with clinically suspected deep vein thrombosis did *not* have this disorder would be a prolonged follow-up on no antithrombotic therapy and suffering no ill effects).

If the report you're reading fails one or more of these three tests you'll need to consider whether it has a fatal flaw that renders its conclusions invalid; if so, it's back to more searching (either now or later; if you haven't enough time, perhaps you can interest a colleague or trainee in taking this on). If the report passes this initial scrutiny and you decide that you can believe its results, but you haven't already carried out the second critical appraisal step of deciding whether these results are impressive, then you can proceed to Section 3b1 on page 118.

Further reading

Jaeschke R, Guyatt G H, Sackett D L for the Evidence-Based Medicine Working Group. Users' guides to the medical literature. VI. How to use an article about a diagnostic test. A: Are the results of the study valid? JAMA 1994; 271: 389–91.

Section 3a2

Is this evidence about prognosis valid?

Clinicians consider questions about prognosis all the time. Sometimes the questions are posed by patients and are quite direct (How long have I got?). At other times the questions are posed by clinicians and are indirect, as when deciding *whether* to treat at all (e.g. an elderly man with chronic lymphocyte leukemia who feels well – would his prognosis be importantly altered if he were left alone until he becomes symptomatic?) or deciding *whether* to screen (e.g. for abdominal aortic aneurysms – what is the fate of the undetected 4 cm aneurysm?). These questions share two elements: a qualitative aspect (Which outcomes could happen?) and a temporal aspect (Over what time period?). In Chapter 1 we showed you how to recognize such questions as being about prognosis and in Chapter 2 we addressed how to find good information about prognosis. In this part of Chapter 3 we'll present a framework for appraising the validity and importance of evidence about prognosis, for use when you tackle situations like the ones above (see Table 3a2.1). We'll consider them in sequence.

The four guides that will help you decide whether some evidence about prognosis is valid are listed in Table 3a2.1. First of all, was a defined, representative sample of patients assembled at a common (usually early) point in the course of their disease? Ideally, the prognosis study you find would include the entire population of patients who ever lived who developed the disease, studied from the instant of its onset. Since this is impossible, you'll want to look at how far from ideal will still tell you what you need to know and you'll do that by finding the methods section (if there isn't one, maybe you're wasting your time on this report!) and reading how the study patients were assembled. You'd want their illness to be defined well enough for you to be clear about it and you'd want the entire spectrum of severity that would occur at that common point to be represented.

Table 3a2.1 Is this evidence about prognosis valid?

1. Was a defined, representative sample of patients assembled at a common (usually early) point in the course of their disease?
2. Was patient follow-up sufficiently long and complete?
3. Were objective outcome criteria applied in a 'blind' fashion?
4. If subgroups with different prognoses are identified:
   - Was there adjustment for important prognostic factors?
   - Was there validation in an independent group of 'test-set' patients?

But when should the 'clock start'? That is, from what point in the disease should patients be followed? If investigators begin tracking outcomes only *after* several patients have already finished their course with the disease, then the outcomes for these patients would never be counted. Some would have recovered quickly, whilst others might have died quickly. So, to avoid missing outcomes by 'starting the clock' too late, you should look to see that study patients were included at a uniformly early time in the disease, ideally when it first becomes clinically manifest, the so-called 'inception cohort'. An exception might be if you wanted to learn about the prognosis of a late stage in the disease (e.g. for clinically manifest coronary heart disease); in this case you'd look for a representative and well-defined sample of patients who were all at a similarly advanced stage (e.g. when they had their first clinical coronary event, not when they first developed elevated coronary risk factors).

Second, was patient follow-up sufficiently long and complete? Ideally, every patient in the inception cohort would be followed over time until they fully recover or one of the disease outcomes occurs. If with short follow-up few study patients have any of the outcomes of interest, you won't have enough to go on when advising your patients. Of course, if after decades of follow-up few adverse events have occurred, this good prognostic result is very useful in reassuring your patient about the future. If you think that the follow-up is too short to have developed a valid picture of the extent of the outcome of your interest, you'd better look for other evidence.

If follow-up was long enough, you still have to worry about patients who entered the study but got lost along the way. Patients are almost always lost to follow-up and their outcomes will be excluded from the study's conclusions about prognosis. Some losses to follow-up are both unavoidable and unrelated to prognosis (e.g. moving away to a better job) and these aren't a cause for worry. But other losses might be because patients die or are too ill to continue follow-up (or lose their independence and move in with family) and the failure to document and report their outcomes will threaten the validity of the report. Short of finding a report that kept track of every patient, how can you judge whether follow-up is 'sufficiently complete'? There is no single answer for all studies, but we offer two suggestions to help you make this judgment. The first is a simple '5 and 20' rule of thumb: fewer than 5% loss probably leads to little bias, greater than 20% loss seriously threatens validity and in-between amounts cause intermediate amounts of trouble. While this may be easy to remember, it may oversimplify for clinical situations in which the outcomes are infrequent.

The second approach uses a 'worst-case' scenario. Imagine a study of prognosis wherein 100 patients enter the study, four die and 16 are lost to follow-up. A 'crude' survival rate would count the four deaths among the 84 with total follow-up, for a death rate of 4.8%, and then report a survival rate of $100\% - 4.8\% = 95.2\%$. But what of the lost 16? Some or all of them might have died too. The latter, 'worst-case' scenario would mean a case-fatality rate of (four known + 16 lost) or 20 out of (84 followed up + 16 lost) or 20/100, that is 20% (four times the observed rate!); note that in order to determine the 'worst-case' scenario you've added the lost patients to both the numerator and denominator of the outcome rate. On the other hand, in the 'best-case' scenario none of the lost 16 would have died, yielding a case-fatality rate of 4 out of (84 + 16) or 4/100, that is 4%; note that in determining the 'best-case' scenario you add the missing cases to just the denominator. While this 'best case' of 4% may not differ much from the observed 4.8%, the 'worst case' of 20% does differ meaningfully and you'd probably judge that this study's follow-up

was not sufficiently complete. By seeing what effect the losses might have on the result you can decide whether a 'worst-case' scenario would change your conclusion about prognosis. If this simple form of 'sensitivity analysis' suggests that losses wouldn't change the result much, then you can judge the follow-up as sufficiently complete.

You can use these first two guides to screen articles about prognosis to find the few worth more of your limited time. If you've answered 'no' to both of the above questions, you can be pretty sure the study will not provide estimates of prognosis that are close to the truth and you ought to start searching for better evidence. If, on the other hand, you've answered 'yes' to both of the above questions, you can be reasonably confident that the study will provide accurate information about prognosis. To be even more sure of this, you should ask the remaining two validity questions in Table 3a2.1.

Were objective outcome criteria applied in a 'blind' fashion? Diseases can affect patients in many important ways; some are easy to spot and some are more subtle. In general, outcomes at both extremes, death or full recovery, are relatively easy to detect and be sure of. In between these extremes are a wide range of outcomes that can be more difficult to detect or confirm and where investigators will have to use judgment in deciding how to count them up. Examples include the degree of disease activity/quiescence, the readiness for return to work and the intensity of residual pain. To minimize the effects of bias, investigators can establish specific criteria that define each possible outcome of the disease and then use these criteria during patient follow-up. You can usually find such outcome criteria in the text, tables, appendices or references in the study. You should satisfy yourself that they are sufficiently objective for confirming the outcomes you're interested in. The occurrence of death is about as objective as you can get, but judging the underlying cause of death is very prone to error (especially when it's based on death certificates) and can be biased unless objective criteria are applied to high-quality clinical evidence.

But even with objective criteria, some bias might creep in if the investigators judging the outcomes also know the

patients' characteristics. To minimize this bias, the authors of the report should have taken precautions so that the investigators making judgments about clinical outcomes were 'blind' to these patients' clinical characteristics and prognostic factors. The more subjective the outcome, the more important such blinding becomes. You should satisfy yourself that blinding was used if it would have been important for the outcomes of interest to you.

The final pair of guides have to do with reports that claim that one subgroup of patients has a different prognosis from others. Such reports are common and for good clinical reason. Often you will want to know whether subgroups of patients have different prognoses (e.g. among patients with non-valvular atrial fibrillation, are those with enlarged left atria at higher risk for stroke than those with normal sized atria?). The first guide here suggests that you look to see whether there was adjustment for other important prognostic factors. That is, reports that address this sort of question should have made sure that these subgroup predictions aren't being distorted by the unequal occurrence of another, powerful prognostic factor (such as would occur if patients with large atria were also more likely to have had prior embolic stroke than patients with normal atria). There are both simple (e.g. stratified analyses displaying the prognoses of patients with large atria separately for those with and without prior embolic stroke) and fancy (e.g. multiple regression analyses that could take into account not only prior embolic stroke but also hypertension, left ventricular function and the like) ways of adjusting for these other important prognostic factors and you should reassure yourself that one or the other has been applied before you tentatively accept the conclusion about a different prognosis for the subgroup of interest.

We say tentatively because there is one final guide to deciding whether a claim that a subgroup has a different prognosis should be accepted as valid. This is the fact that the statistics of determining subgroup prognoses are all about prediction, not explanation. They are indifferent to whether the prognostic factor is physiologically logical (in our running example, left atrial size) or biologically nonsensical (whether the patient's navel is concave (an 'innie') or convex (an 'outie'). These prognostic factors can be demographic (such as age, gender, socioeconomic status), disease specific (such as extent of disease, degree of test abnormality) or comorbid (presence or absence of many other conditions). Keep in mind that these prognostic factors need not cause the outcome; they need only be associated with its development strongly enough to predict it.

For this reason, the first time a prognostic factor is identified, there is no guarantee it isn't the result of a random, non-causal 'quirk' in its distribution between patients with different prognoses; for that reason, the initial patient group in which it was identified is called a 'training set'. As you might imagine, if this initial study carried out a multivariate analysis looking for potential prognostic factors, they'd be very likely to find at least a few, just on the basis of chance (and most investigators would be imaginative enough to suggest logical explanations for them). Because of this risk of spurious, chance nomination of prognostic factors, you should seek its confirmation in a report of a second, independent group (called a 'test set') of patients. The best evidence for this is finding a statement (in the methods section) of a prestudy intention to examine this specific possible prognostic factor (based on its appearance in a training set). If that second, independent study also identifies the prognostic factor, you can feel much more confident that the evidence about it is valid.

If your evidence flunks these tests for validity, we're afraid it's back to searching, either now (if you still have time) or at a later session. If, on a happier note, you decide that the evidence you've found about a prognostic factor is valid and you haven't already decided whether it's also important, you can take that consideration up in Section 3b2 on page 129.

Further reading

Laupacis A, Wells G, Richardson W S, Tugwell P for the Evidence-Based Medicine Working Group. Users' guides to the medical literature. V. How to use an article about prognosis. JAMA 1994; 272: 234-7.

Section 3a3

Is this evidence about a treatment valid?

Having found some possibly useful evidence about therapy, you have to decide where to start in its critical appraisal. On the one hand, you could start here in Section 3a3, with an appraisal of its validity (arguing that if it's not valid, who cares whether it appears to show a big effect?). On the other, you could go right to determining its importance in Section 3b3 (arguing that if the evidence doesn't suggest a possibly useful clinical impact, who cares if it's valid?). Begin with either and then pick up the other. This section will help you to quickly and critically appraise evidence about therapy for its closeness to the truth. This can be done by asking some simple questions and often you'll find their answers in an abstract that accompanies the evidence. Table 3a3.1 lists these questions for reports of individual therapeutic trials, but since these can best be interpreted in the context of all other trials on the same topic, Table 3a3.2 summarizes guides for assessing evidence that has combined the results of several trials into an overview or systematic review (when a systematic review uses special statistical methods for combining the results of several studies, we call it a meta-analysis). Alternatively, you may encounter (or have tracked down) an economic analysis, which is a more complex method that compares therapeutic alternatives from a broader perspective (including those of health managers or even society as a whole) and tries to offer or provide treatments in the way that best uses scarce resources such as hospital beds, drugs, operating time, clinicians and money. Questions pertinent to deciding whether you should believe an economic analysis appear in Table 3a3.3. Finally, and building on the earlier section on diagnosis, we'll give you a brief description of how to decide whether to believe evidence on the effects of therapy when it is formulated into a clinical decision analysis; rules for deciding whether to believe their results are described in Section 3a3.4.

Table 3a3.1 Are the results of this single study valid?

The main questions to answer:
1 Was the assignment of patients to treatments randomized? and was the randomization list concealed?
2 Were all patients who entered the trial accounted for at its conclusion? and were they analyzed in the groups to which they were randomized?

And some finer points to address:
1 Were patients and clinicians kept 'blind' to which treatment was being received?
2 Aside from the experimental treatment, were the groups treated equally?
3 Were the groups similar at the start of the trial?

When several randomized trials of the same treatment for the same condition have been carried out, we think you'll agree that an overview which systematically reviews and combines all of them would give you a better answer than a critical appraisal of just one of them. For that reason, we suggested back in Chapter 2 that you always start your search for useful clinical articles on just about any topic by looking for systematic reviews. However, because systematic reviews assess their component trials individually (and, as you can see in Table 3a3.2, you want to be sure that they've done that in a valid way) and since at this point in history you're much more likely to find individual trials than systematic reviews, we'll begin with the individual trial.

Is the evidence from this randomized trial valid?

We'll begin with two important questions:

1. Was the assignment of patients to treatments randomized and was the randomization schedule concealed?

When deciding whether the evidence from a randomized trial is valid, the most important question to ask (and frequently the quickest question to answer) is: Was the assignment of patients to treatments randomized? That is, was some method analogous to tossing a coin* used to assign patients to treatments (with the treatment you're interested in given if the coin landed 'heads' and a conventional, 'control' or placebo† treatment given if the coin landed 'tails')? The reason for insisting on random allocation to treatments is that this comes closer than any other research design to creating groups of patients at the start of the trial who are identical in their risk of the events you're hoping to prevent. It does this in two, related ways. First, the coin toss balances the groups for prognostic factors (such as disease severity or other predictors of especially good or bad prognosis) which, if they were unevenly distributed between treatment groups, could exaggerate, cancel or even counteract the effects of therapy.‡ If they exaggerated the apparent effects of an otherwise ineffectual treatment, the effects of their imbalance could lead to the false-positive conclusion that the treatment was useful when it was not. And if they cancelled or counteracted the effects of a really efficacious treatment, the effects of their imbalance could lead to the false-negative conclusions that a useful treatment was useless or even harmful. Random allocation balances the treatment groups for these and other prognostic factors, even if we don't yet understand the disorder well enough to know what they are!

The second, related benefit of random allocation is that, if it is concealed from the clinicians who are entering patients into the trial, they will be unaware of which treatment the next patient will receive and they can't either consciously or unconsciously distort the balance between the groups being compared. So you want to be sure that both of these standards are met. Usually it's easy to tell whether a study was

* In practice, this coin tossing is done by special computer programs, but the principle is exactly the same.
† A placebo is a treatment that is so similar in appearance, taste, etc. that the patient ('single-blind') or the clinician or both ('double-blind') are unable to distinguish it from the active treatment.
‡ 'Confounder' is a technical name for these sorts of patient characteristics that are extraneous to the question posed, could cause the clinical events we are trying to prevent with the treatment and might be unevenly distributed between the treatment groups. And although there are other ways of avoiding confounding (exclusion, stratified sampling, matching, stratified analysis, standardization and multivariate modelling), they all demand that you already know what the confounder is.

randomized, because it's something to be proud of and that term often appears in the title and almost always in the abstract. On the other hand, it's not often stated whether the randomization list was concealed, but if randomization occurred by telephone or by some system that was at a distance from where patients were being entered into the trial, you can be comfortable about this. If randomization wasn't concealed, this tends to lead to patients with more favourable prognoses being given the experimental treatment, exaggerating the apparent benefits of therapy and perhaps even leading to the false-positive conclusion that the treatment is efficacious when it is not.

If you find that the study was not randomized, we'd suggest that you stop reading it and go on to the next article. Only if you can't find any randomized trials should you come back and have another go at it. But if the only evidence you have about a treatment is from non-randomized studies, you are in a bind and have five options:

1. Check Chapter 2 again or get help in doing another literature search to see if you missed any randomized trials of the candidate therapy.

2. See whether the treatment effect is simply so huge that you can't imagine it could be a false-positive study (this usually happens only when the prognosis is uniformly awful and is a very rare situation). As a check, ask several colleagues whether they consider the candidate therapy so likely to be efficacious that they'd consider it unethical to randomize a patient like yours into a study of it that includes a no-treatment or placebo group.*

3. Conversely, if the non-randomized study concluded that the treatment was useless or harmful, then it is usually safe to accept that conclusion (since, as described above, false-negative conclusions from non-randomized studies are less likely than false-positive ones).

4. Consider whether an 'N-of-1' trial would make sense to you and your patient (they are described on page 173).

* This is the 'convincing non-experimental evidence' category used in the audits of clinical care reported on page 3 (the A-team study).

5. Try some other treatment or simply provide supportive care.

2. Were all patients who entered the trial accounted for at its conclusion and were they analysed in the groups to which they were randomized?

Having satisfied yourself that the trial really was randomized, you can then match the number of patients who entered the trial with the number accounted for at its conclusion. Ideally, these numbers will be identical, for lost patients could have had events that would change the conclusion. If, for example, patients on the experimental treatment dropped out and had adverse outcomes, their absence from the analysis would lead it to overestimate the efficacy of that treatment. What's an acceptable loss? To be sure of a trial's conclusion, its authors should be able to take all patients who were lost along the way, assign them the 'worst-case' outcomes (that is, assume that everyone lost from the group whose remaining members fared better had a bad outcome and assume that everyone lost from the group whose remaining members fared worse had a rosy outcome) and still be able to support their original conclusion. It would be unusual for a trial to withstand a worst-case analysis if it lost more than 20% of its patients and journals like *Evidence-Based Medicine* won't publish trials with <80% follow-up.

Because anything that happens after randomization can affect the chances that a patient in a trial has an event, it's important that all patients (even those who fail to take their medicine or accidentally or intentionally receive the wrong treatment) are analysed in the groups to which they were randomized. This is an essential prerequisite for valid evidence about the effects of therapy. For example, it has repeatedly been shown that patients who do and don't take their study medicine have very different outcomes, even when the study medicine they have been prescribed is a placebo! The correct form of analysis, in which patients are analysed in the groups to which they were assigned, is called an 'intention to treat' analysis.

There are three less important questions to ask when you are trying to decide whether a randomized trial has produced valid evidence:

1. Were patients and clinicians kept 'blind' to which treatment was being received?
2. Aside from the experimental treatment, were the groups treated equally?
3. Were the groups similar at the start of the trial?

If you decide that the study really was randomized, follow-up was virtually complete and patients were analyzed in the groups to which they'd been randomized, you can look for some other features that provide even greater assurance that you can believe its results. If, for example, it was a pharmacological trial in which patients received either a tablet containing the active drug or an identical-appearing (in size, shape, colour, taste, etc.) tablet of pharmacologically inert ingredients (a placebo), then it would be possible to keep both patients and clinicians blind* as to which treatment was received and neither the patient's reporting of symptoms nor the clinician's interpretation of them would be influenced by their hunches about whether the treatment was efficacious. Another advantage of the double-blind method is that it prevents patients and their clinicians from adding any additional treatments (or 'cointerventions') to just one of the groups. When patients and their clinicians can't be kept blind (as in surgical trials), often it is possible to have other, blinded clinicians come in and assess clinical records (purged of any mention of treatment) or make special outcome measurements. And finally, you can double-check to see whether randomization was effective by looking to see whether patients were similar at the start of the trial (most trials display this in the first table of their results).

Whether the results of an individual trial are important is considered in Section 3b3 on page 133.

* When patients don't know their treatment but their doctors do (as when the active drug causes a clearcut sign such as bradycardia), the trial is called 'single blind'. When both are blind, it is called 'double blind'.

Is the evidence from this systematic review valid?

Having shown you how to decide whether to believe the results of a single trial, let's now turn to how you can decide whether to believe the results of an overview of several trials. The key questions you need to answer are in Table 3a3.2.

Table 3a3.2 Are the results of this systematic review valid?

1. Is it an overview of randomized trials of the treatment you're interested in?
2. Does it include a methods section that describes:
   a. finding and including all the relevant trials?
   b. assessing their individual validity?
3. Were the results consistent from study to study?

1. Is it a systematic review of randomized trials of the treatment you're interested in?

This first question asks whether you are sure that the treatment is the same as the one you're considering and immediately asking whether the overview is combining reports of studies carried out at the same, most powerful level of evidence that we've been discussing here, the randomized trial. Systematic reviews of non-randomized studies of therapy simply compound the problems of individually misleading trials and the same warnings apply. Moreover, some overviews combine randomized and non-randomized studies and unless the authors have provided separate information on the subset of randomized trials, you shouldn't trust them either.

2. Does it include a methods section that describes: (a) finding and including all the relevant trials; (b) assessing their individual validity?

You should see whether the overview report includes a methods section that describes how they found all the relevant trials and how they assessed their individual validity. Let's take these three elements one by one. First, because performing an overview is performing research (it involves posing a question, identifying a population and drawing a sample, making measurements, analyzing them and drawing

conclusions), it should be carried out and reported like research. If you don't find a methods section, be very wary of believing its results; maybe its only useful part will be its bibliography of individual trials for you to study as above. Second, if the overview has a methods section it should describe how its authors tracked down and included all the trials that were relevant to this treatment. This is no easy task. The standard bibliographic databases described in Chapter 2, good as they are, fail to correctly label up to half of the published trials and 'negative' trials (that conclude that treatment is not efficacious) are less likely to be submitted for publication, leading an overview of those that are published to overestimate the treatment's efficacy. Signs that the overviewers did a good job are positive when they report at least some hand searching of the most relevant journals (for miscoded trials) and especially when they report contacting the authors of published trials (who often will know about unpublished ones). Third, you should look for a statement of how they decided whether the individual trials in their overview were scientifically sound, using criteria like those in Table 3a3.1. Finally, because these last two steps of deciding which trials to include in the overview involve a lot of judgment calls, you should be especially reassured when you find that two or more investigators carried out these tasks independent of each other and achieved good agreement about their judgments.

3. Were the results consistent from study to study?

It stands to reason that we are more likely to believe an overview when the results of all the trials in it show a treatment effect going in the same direction. Although we shouldn't expect each of them to show exactly the same degree of efficacy (that is, we should be comfortable with a certain amount of quantitative difference in the trial results), we would be concerned if we found some trials in an overview confidently concluding a beneficial effect of the treatment and other trials confidently concluding no benefit or a harmful effect. Such a qualitative difference in the effects of treatment (which also goes by the name of heterogeneity), unless it can be explained to your satisfaction (such

Table 3a4.1 Are the results of this harm study valid?

1. Were there clearly defined groups of patients, similar in all important ways other than exposure to the treatment?
2. Were treatment exposures and clinical outcomes measured in the same way in both groups?
3. Was the follow-up of study patients complete and long enough?
4. Do the results satisfy some 'diagnostic tests for causation'?
 • Is it clear that the exposure preceded the onset of the outcome?
 • Is there a dose-response gradient?
 • Is there positive evidence from a 'dechallenge-rechallenge' study?
 • Is the association consistent from study to study?
 • Does the association make biological sense?

Section 3a4

Is this evidence about harm valid?

You must frequently make judgments on whether a treatment is harming or has harmed a patient. Many admissions to acute general hospitals are the result of adverse drug reactions and reactions to diagnostic and therapeutic maneuvers are judged to befall one-fifth to one-third of patients after they are admitted. On the other hand, even clinical pharmacologists disagree about whether a given patient has had an adverse drug reaction and the fact that an adverse reaction occurred *during* a treatment is insufficient evidence that it occurred *because* of that treatment.

Faced with a problem that is pandemic yet controvertible, clinicians must equip themselves to answer two related questions:

1. Does this drug (or operation or other treatment) cause that adverse effect in *some* patients? And, if so:
2. Did this drug (or operation or other treatment) cause that adverse effect in *this particular* patient?

This section will deal with the first question and the second question will be addressed in Section 4.4.

Because this assessment can be viewed as addressing a general question of *causation*, it benefits from what has been learned about asking and answering such questions in classical epidemiology. The four guides for deciding whether to believe the claim that a treatment harms some patients are summarized in Table 3a4.1, and we'll consider them in sequence.

1. Were there clearly defined groups of patients, similar in all important ways other than exposure to the treatment?

Because the 'threats to validity' are different for different sorts of studies, you'll have to spend just a little time sorting them out. Suppose you wanted to decide whether fenoterol (a beta-agonist used to treat asthma) sometimes (albeit

rarely) caused the death of its users. You could look for and find four different sorts of studies and all of them can be illustrated by reference to Table 3a4.2. First, you could look for a randomized trial in which asthma patients were assigned, by a system analogous to tossing a coin, to receive fenoterol (the top row in Table 3a4.2, whose total is **a+b**)

		Adverse Outcome		Totals
		Present (Case)	Absent (Control)	
Exposed to the treatment	Yes (Cohort)	a	b	a+b
	No (Cohort)	c	d	c+d
	Totals	a+c	b+d	a+b+c+d

Table 3a4.2 Different ways of finding out whether a treatment sometimes causes harm

---

as by differences in patients or in doses or durations of treatment), should lead you to be very cautious about believing any overall conclusion about efficacy in all patients and you'd hope to see your caution expressed in the conclusions of the overview.

Whether the results of an overview are important is considered in Section 3b3 on page 133.

or some comparison treatment or placebo (the bottom row, whose total is **c+d**). Since the randomization would make them similar for all other features that would cause their deaths, you'd be pretty likely to judge any statistically significant increase in deaths among fenoterol recipients (cell **a**) as valid. Trouble is, if fenoterol causes only one extra death per 1000 users, you'd have to find an awfully big trial to show a clear excess among fenoterol-treated asthmatics. As it happens, if a drug causes an adverse reaction once per x patients who receive it (say, once per 1000), to be 95% certain to see at least one adverse reaction you need to follow 3x patients (in this example, 3000). For that reason, you usually can't find the most valid data on harm from individual randomized trials and if you can't find a systematic review with a large enough total number of patients to suffice, you'll have to work with non-experimental evidence.

The next most powerful design is also conducted along the rows of Table 3a4.2, but this time the groups of patients (called 'cohorts') who are (**a+b**) and are not (**c+d**) exposed to the treatment are formed not by random allocation, but by the decisions of clinicians and patients to have some of them ('exposed') receive the treatment and others ('unexposed') not receive it. These cohorts are then followed to determine which and how many of them develop the bad outcome (**a** or **c**). As you can see, there is no reason why these cohorts should be otherwise perfectly identical to each other and plenty of reason for them to be quite different (e.g. sicker patients who are more likely to have adverse outcomes might be more likely to be offered a 'last-ditch' treatment). Since there may be strong links between the prognosis of patients and the probability that they will be offered and accept a treatment (sometimes called 'confounding'), the analyses of these cohort analytic studies are difficult and often involve trying to correct for known confounders (such as disease severity) by statistical methods (all the way from simply comparing outcomes within patients with different degrees of severity to quite fancy multivariate analyses). But we can't adjust for what we don't yet know about the determinants of disease outcomes, so you have to be cautious in interpreting cohort studies.

And for rare or late complications of treatments, not even cohort studies are big enough and often you'll have to rely on studies conducted vertically in Table 3a4.2 by assembling cases (**a+c**) who already have the bad outcome, assembling a second group of 'controls' (**b+d**) who don't have the bad outcome and tracking back in their histories or records to determine the proportions of each group who were exposed to the suspect treatment (**a** or **b**): a case-control study. This is, in fact, what was done in trying to sort out the fenoterol problem: asthma deaths (cases) were compared with living asthma patients (controls) for their use of fenoterol and these comparisons were 'adjusted' for the severity of their asthma. The problem of confounding (of prognosis with exposure) is even worse in case-control studies than in cohort studies, for often it is impossible to measure the confounders among cases, even if they are known.* For this reason, case-control studies are viewed with even greater caution than cohort studies. Finally, you may find reports of one or a few patients who developed the bad outcome while under treatment (just cell **a**). If the outcome is unique and dramatic (phocomelia in children born to women who took thalidomide) case reports and case series may be enough, but usually they simply point to the need for the other types of studies.

As with other issues in clinical and health care, the best evidence on adverse effects will come from a systematic review of all the relevant studies and these should always be your primary targets when searching for the best external evidence. Systematic reviews of randomized trials or cohort studies may possess sufficiently large numbers of patients to identify even rare adverse effects. Whether appraising a systematic review or an individual study, you'll need to take into account how it assembled and assessed its members and now that you've learned how to recognize the sort of study you're reading, you can apply the guides in Table 3a4.1:

1. From the foregoing discussion, it's clear why you want the report to describe clearly defined groups of

patients, similar in all important ways other than exposure to the treatment (to get rid of confounders).

2. Moreover, it makes sense that you should place greater confidence in reports of studies in which treatment exposures and clinical outcomes were measured the same ways in both groups (you'd not want one group studied more exhaustively than the other, because this would lead to reporting a greater occurrence of exposure or outcome in the more intensively studied group).

3. Furthermore, in a report concluding that the treatment was innocent, you'd want the follow-up of study patients to have been complete and long enough for the bad effects to have had time to reveal themselves.

4. Finally, you'd want to determine whether the association met at least some common-sense 'diagnostic tests for causation':

● you'd want to be sure that the exposure (say, use of a psychotropic drug) preceded the onset of the bad outcome (say, behavior ending in suicide), and wasn't just a 'marker' (say, of depression) that it was already underway;

● the validity of a claim that a treatment causes an adverse outcome receives a real boost when increasing doses or durations of the treatment are associated with increasing frequency or severity of the adverse outcome: a 'dose-response' effect;

● the validity of a claim is also boosted if there is documentation that the adverse effect decreased or disappeared when the treatment was withdrawn ('dechallenge') and worsened or reappeared when the treatment was reintroduced ('rechallenge');

● if you are fortunate enough to have found a systematic review of the question, you can determine whether the association of exposure to the suspect treatment and the adverse outcome is consistent from study to study. When it is, your confidence in the validity of the association deserves to increase;

● finally, it boosts your confidence when the association makes biological sense.

---

* Dead patients tell no tales and information about exposures to lethal treatments may perish with their victims.

If the report fails to meet the first three minimum standards, you're better off abandoning it and continuing your search. On the other hand, if you're satisfied that the report meets these minimum guides, you can decide whether the relation between exposure and outcome is strong and convincing enough for you to need to do something about it and that's discussed in Section 3b4.

Further reading

Levine M, Walter S D, Lee H, Haines T, Holbrook A, Moyer V for the Evidence-Based Medicine Working Group. Users' guides to the medical literature: IV. How to use an article about harm. JAMA 1994; 271: 1615–19.

Section 3b1

Is this evidence about a diagnostic test important?

In deciding whether the evidence about a diagnostic test is important, we will focus on a modern way of thinking about diagnosis that takes into account both components of evidence-based medicine: your individual clinical expertise and the best external evidence. The former is your prior assessment of diagnostic possibilities before you do the test ('prior or pretest probabilities') and the latter is the ability of the test to distinguish patients with and without the target disorder (both the oldfashioned concepts of sensitivity and specificity and the newfangled and more powerful ideas around likelihood ratios). We'll show you how to combine these two elements of EBM to refine your estimates of the target disorder ('posterior or post-test probabilities') and make the diagnosis. Diagnostic tests that produce big changes from pretest to post-test probabilities are important and likely to be useful to you in your practice.

Where do these pretest probabilities come from? Usually they are derived from your own accumulating clinical experience, specific for the setting in which you work and the sorts of patients you see. As a result, pretest probabilities for the same target disorder can vary widely between and within countries and between primary, secondary and tertiary care. We have summarized some published pretest probabilities in Table 3b1.1 and more are available from our Website.

Suppose that you're working up a patient with anemia and think that the probability that they have iron deficiency anemia is 50%; that is, the odds are about 50–50 that it's due to iron deficiency. When you present the patient to your boss, you ask for an educational prescription to determine the usefulness of performing a serum ferritin on your patient as a means of detecting iron deficiency anemia. Suppose further that, in filling your prescription, you find a systematic

Table 3b1.1 Some pretest probabilities

Patient problem	Clinical setting	Target disorder	Pretest probability
Melena in a 50-year-old man who drinks 25 units of alcohol a week but has no stigmata of liver disease	Emergency room in North America	Varices	5%
		Benign ulcer	55%
		Gastritis	40%
Symptomless 60-69-year-olds	Primary care	Undiagnosed colon cancer: all patients positive family history	0.5% 1.5%
Symptomless Woman 30-39 y/o 60-69 y/o	Primary care	≥ 75% stenosis of one or more coronary arteries	0.3% 6%
Man			2% 12%
Non-anginal chest pain Woman 30-39 y/o 60-69 y/o			1% 19%
Man 30-39 y/o 60-69 y/o			5% 28%
Atypical angina Woman 30-39 y/o 60-69 y/o			4% 54%
Man 30-39 y/o 60-69 y/o			22% 67%
Typical angina pectoris Woman 30-39 y/o 60-69 y/o			26% 91%
Man 30-39 y/o 60-69 y/o			70% 94%
Symptomless 50 y/o with a solitary pulmonary nodule	Primary care	Cancer for any nodules For 3 cm nodules	50% 65%

To find more examples, and to nominate additions to the databank of pretest probabilities, refer to this textbook's Website at: http://cebm.jr2.ox.ac.uk/

review of several studies of this diagnostic test (evaluated against the reference standard of a bone marrow stain for iron), decide that it is valid (based on the guides in Tables 3a3.2 and 3a1.1), and find their results as shown in Table 3b1.2. By the time you've tracked down and studied the external evidence, your patient's serum ferritin comes back at 60 mmol/L. How should you put all this together?

As you can see from Table 3b1.2, your patient's result places them in the top row of the table, either in cell **a** or cell **b**. From that fact you would conclude several things: first, you'd note that 90% of patients with iron deficiency have serum ferritins in the same range as your patient, (**a/(a+c)**), and that property, the proportion of patients with the target disorder who have positive test results, is called sensitivity.

Table 3b1.2 Results of a systematic review of serum ferritin as a diagnostic test for iron deficiency anemia

		Target disorder (iron deficiency anemia)		Totals
		Present	Absent	
Diagnostic test result (serum ferritin)	Positive (<65 mmol/L	731 a	270 b	1001 a+b
	Negative (≥65 mmol/L	78 c	1500 d	1578 c+d
Totals		809 a+c	1770 b+d	2579 a+b+c+d

Sensitivity = **a/(a+c)** = 731/809 = 90%
Specificity = **d/(b+d)** = 1500/1770 = 85%
LR+ = sens/(1–spec) = 90%/15% = 6
LR– = (1–sens)/spec = 10%/85% = 0.12
Positive predictive value = **a/(a+b)** = 731/1001 = 73%
Negative predictive value = **d/(c+d)** = 1500/1578 = 95%
Prevalence = **(a+c)/(a+b+c+d)** = 809/2579 = 32%
Pretest odds = prevalence/(1–prevalence) = 31%/69% = 0.45
Post-test odds = pretest odds × likelihood ratio
Post-test probability = post-test odds/(post-test odds +1)

And you might also note that only 15% of patients with other causes for their anemia have results in the same range as your patient,* which means that your patient's result would be about six times as likely (90% / 15%) to be seen in someone with, as opposed to someone without, iron deficiency anemia and that's called the likelihood ratio for a positive test result. Furthermore, since you thought ahead of time (before you had the result of the serum ferritin) that your patient's odds of iron deficiency were 50–50, that's called a pretest odds of 1:1 and, as you can see from the formulae towards the bottom of Table 3b1.2, you can multiply that pretest odds of 1 by the likelihood ratio of 6 to get the post-test odds of iron deficiency anemia after the test: 1×6 = 6. Since, like most clinicians, you may be more comfortable thinking in terms of probabilities than odds, this post-test odds of 6:1 converts (as you can see at the bottom of Table 3b1.2) to a post-test probability of 6/(6+1) = 6/7 = 86%. So it looks like you've made the diagnosis and this diagnostic test looks worthwhile.

(To check yourself out on these calculations, try the same ferritin result for a patient who, like those in the table, has a pretest odds of 0.47;† you'll know you did it right if you wind up with an answer identical to its equivalent, the positive predictive value.)

Extremely high values of sensitivity and specificity are useful, but not for the reasons you may think.‡ When a test has a very high sensitivity (such as the loss of retinal vein pulsation in increased intracranial pressure), a negative result (the presence of pulsation) effectively rules out the diagnosis (of raised intracranial pressure) and one of our clinical clerks suggested that we apply the mnemonic SnNout to such findings (when a sign has a high *Sn*sitivity, a *N*egative result rules *out* the diagnosis). Similarly, when a sign has a very high specificity (such as a fluid wave for ascites), a positive result effectively rules in the diagnosis (of ascites); not surprisingly, our clinical clerks call such a finding a SpPin (when a sign has a high *Sp*ecificity, a *P*ositive result rules *in* the diagnosis). We've listed some SpPins and SnNouts in Table 3b1.3 and have generated a longer list on our Website.

* The complement of this proportion is called specificity and it describes the proportion of patients who do not have the target disorder who have negative or normal test results, **d/(b+d)**.
† The post-test odds are 0.45 × 6 = 2.7 and the post-test probability is 2.7/3.7 = 73%. Note that this is identical to the positive predictive value.
‡ On first encounter, most learners think that tests with high sensitivity rule in diagnoses and tests with high specificity rule them out; the reverse is the case.

Although the serum ferritin determination looks impressive when viewed in terms of its sensitivity (90%) and specificity (85%), the newer way of expressing its accuracy with likelihood ratios reveals its even greater power and, in this particular example, shows how we can be misled by the fact that the old sensitivity–specificity approach restricts us to just two levels (positive and negative) of the test result. Most test results, like serum ferritin, can be divided into several levels and in Table 3b1.4 we show you a particularly useful way of dividing test results into five levels. When this is done, one extreme level of the test result can be shown to rule in the diagnosis and in this case you can SpPin 59% of the patients with iron deficiency anemia, despite the unimpressive sensitivity (59%) that would have been achieved if the ferritin results had been split at this level. Likelihood ratios of 10 or more, when applied to pretest probabilities of 33% or more (.33/.67 = pretest odds of 0.5) will generate post-test probabilities of 5/6 = 83% or more. Moreover, the other extreme level can SnNout 75% of those who do not have iron deficiency anemia (again despite a not very impressive specificity of 75%). Likelihood ratios of 0.1 or less, when applied to pretest probabilities of 33% or less (.33/.67 = pretest odds of 0.5) will generate post-test probabilities of 0.05/1.05 = 5% or less. Two other intermediate levels can move a 50% prior probability (pretest odds of 1:1) to the useful but not usually diagnostic post-test probabilities of 4.8/5.8 = 83% and 0.39/1.39 = 28%. And one indeterminate level in the middle (containing about 10% of both sorts of patients) can be seen to be uninformative, with a likelihood ratio of 1. We've shown the effects of these sorts of likelihood ratios on these sorts of pretest probabilities in Table 3b1.5.

Table 3b1.3 Some SpPins and SnNouts

Target disorder	SpPin (& specificity) [presence rules in the target disorder]	SnNout (& sensitivity) [absence rules out the target disorder]
Ascites (by imaging or tap)*	Fluid wave (92%)	History of ankle swelling (93%)
Pleural effusion†	Auscultatory percussion note loud and sharp (100%)	Auscultatory percussion note soft and/or dull (96%)
Increased intracranial pressure (by CAT scan or direct measurement)‡		Loss of spontaneous retinal vein pulsation (100%)
Cancer as a cause of lower back pain (by further investigation)§		Age >50 or cancer history or unexplained weight loss or failure of conservative therapy (100%)
Sinusitis (by further investigation)¶		Maxillary toothache or purulent nasal secretion or poor response to nasal decongestants or abnormal transillumination or history of coloured nasal discharge
Alcohol abuse or dependency**	Yes to ≥3 of the CAGE questions (99.8%)	
Splenomegaly (by imaging)††	Positive percussion (Nixon method) and palpation	
Non-urgent cause for dizziness‡‡		Positive head-hanging test and either vertigo or vomiting (94%)

To find more examples, and to nominate additions to the databank of SpPins and SnNouts, refer to this textbook's Website at: http://cebm.jr2.ox.ac.uk/

* JAMA 1992; 267: 2645–8.
† J Gen Int Med 1994; 9: 71–4.
‡ Arch Neurol 1978; 35: 37–40.
§ JAMA 1992; 268: 760–5.
* JAMA 1993; 270: 1242–6.
** Amer J Med 1987; 82: 231–5.
†† JAMA 1993; 270: 2218–21.
‡‡ JAMA 1994; 271: 385–8.

Table 3b1.4 The usefulness of five levels of a diagnostic test result

Diagnostic test result	Serum ferritin (mmol/L)	Target disorder present		Target disorder absent		Likelihood ratio	Diagnostic impact
		Number	%	Number	%		
Very positive	<15	474	59%	20	1.1%	52	Rule in SpPin
Moderately positive	15–34	175	22%	79	4.5%	4.8	Intermediate high
Neutral	35–64	82	10%	171	10%	1	Indeterminate
Moderately negative	65–94	30	3.7%	168	9.5%	0.39	Intermediate low
Extremely negative	≥95	48	5.9%	1332	75%	0.08	Rule out SnNout
		809	100%	1770	100%		

Table 3b1.5 Some post-test probabilities generated by five levels of a diagnostic test result

Likelihood ratio	Post-test probability of the target disorder for different pretest probabilities						Diagnostic impact
	Pre-test 5%	Pre-test 10%	Pre-test 20%	Pre-test 30%	Pre-test 50%	Pre-test 70%	
Very positive 10	34%	53%	71%	81%	91%	96%	Rule in SpPin
Moderately positive 3	14%	25%	43%	56%	75%	88%	Intermediate high
Neutral 1	5%	10%	20%	30%	50%	70%	Indeterminate
Moderately negative 0.3	1.5%	3.2%	7%	11%	23%	41%	Intermediate low
Extremely negative 0.1	0.5%	1%	2.5%	4%	9%	19%	Rule out SnNout

Finally, there's an easier way of manipulating all these probability↔odds calculations and a nomogram for doing so appears as Figure 3b1.1 and in the pocket cards that come with this book. You can check out your understanding of this nomogram by replicating the results in Table 3b1.5.

To your surprise (we reckon!) your patient's test result generates an indeterminate likelihood ratio of only 1 and the test which you thought might be very useful, based on the sensitivity and specificity way of looking at things, really hasn't been helpful in moving you toward the diagnosis, so you'll have to think about other tests (including perhaps the reference standard of a bone marrow examination) to sort this out.

More and more reports of diagnostic tests are providing multilevel likelihood ratios as measures of their accuracy. When they only report sensitivity and specificity, you can sometimes find a table with more levels and generate your own set of likelihood ratios or you can find a scatter plot (of test results versus diagnoses) that is good enough for you to be able to split into levels. Or, if all you have is sensitivity and specificity, you can generate likelihood ratios from them by reference to the formulae in Table 3b1.2 (the likelihood ratio for a positive test result = LR+ = sensitivity/[1-specificity] and the likelihood ratio for a negative test result = LR− = [1−sensitivity]/specificity).

Some reports into the accuracy of diagnostic tests go beyond even likelihood ratios and one of them deserves mention here. This extension considers multiple diagnostic tests as a cluster or sequence of tests for a given target disorder. These multiple results can be presented in different ways, either as clusters of positive/negative results or as multivariate scores, and in either case they can be ranked and handled just like other multilevel likelihood ratios.

In any event, having decided that a diagnostic test produces important changes from pretest to post-test probabilities, you might want to study the final issue, described in Section 4.1, of how to integrate the results of this critical appraisal with your individual clinical expertise and apply the results to your own patient (but if you jumped to this second step without first determining whether the evidence about this diagnostic test was valid, you'd better go back to Section 3a1 first!).

Further reading

Sackett D L, Haynes R B, Guyatt G H, Tugwell P. Clinical epidemiology: a basic science for clinical medicine, 2nd edn. Little, Brown, Boston, 1991. Chapter 4 (for interpreting diagnostic tests).

Jaeschke R, Guyatt G H, Sackett D L for the Evidence-Based Medicine Working Group. Users' guides to the medical literature. VI. How to use an article about a diagnostic test. A. Are the results of the study valid? JAMA 1994; 271: 389–91. B. What are the results and will they help me in caring for my patients? JAMA 1994; 271: 703–7.

Nomogram for interpreting diagnostic test result

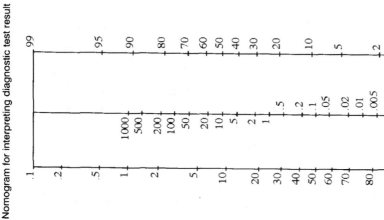

Figure 3b1.1 A likelihood ratio nomogram. Adapted from Fagan T J 1975 Nomogram for Bayes's Theorem (c). New England Journal of Medicine 293: 257

Section 3b2

Is this evidence about prognosis important?

Guides for making this decision appear in Table 3b2.1. First, how likely are the outcomes over time? Diseases usually have more than a single outcome of interest and these can occur in several combinations and at different times following the onset of the disease. Thus, for each important disease outcome, you should examine the article to see how likely each of these outcomes is over time. Typically they are reported as percentage survival at a particular point in time (such as 1-year or 5-year survival rates) and as survival curves of various kinds. Another form of result, common in cancer studies, is the median survival, indicating the length of follow-up by which 50% of the study sample have died. The more numerous the outcome possibilities and the more variable the timing of these outcomes are, the more complex such results can be.

Figure 3b2.1 illustrates some different patterns of prognosis, each leading to different conclusions about prognosis. They are presented in the most frequent format used to describe prognosis, a survival curve that depicts, at each point in time, the proportion (often expressed as a %) of the original study population who have NOT yet had an outcome event.* In panel A, virtually no patients have had events by the end of the study, so either the prognosis is very good (in which case the study is very useful to you) or the study is too short (in which case it's not very useful!). Panels B, C and D depict a serious disease, with only

* How such survival curves are constructed is not described in detail in this book, so don't look for it! In brief, it is done by some clever methods that combine the results from patients who have been followed for just short periods of time as well as long ones and who have had outcomes occur early, late or not at all. Often the strategy used here is a 'life table' method, if you want to look it up.

Table 3b2.1 Is this evidence about prognosis important?

1. How likely are the outcomes over time?
2. How precise are the prognostic estimates?

20% of patients surviving at 1 year; you could tell such patients, then, that their chances of surviving for a year are 20%. Note, however, that the shapes of these curves are quite different, so that the median survival (by which time half of them have succumbed) is 9 months for the disorder described in panel B but only 3 months for the disorder described in panel C. The survival pattern is a steady, uniform decline only in panel D and we hope you can see why the best answer to 'How much time have I got, doc?' often is the time at which half the study patients have died (or suffered some other event of interest); this is called the median survival.

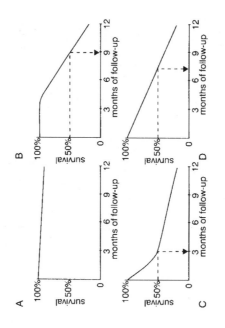

Figure 3b2.1 Prognosis shown as survival curves. Panel A: Good prognosis (or too short a study!). Panel B: Good prognosis early, then worsening, with a median survival of 9 months. Panel C: Bad prognosis early, then better, with a median survival of 3 months. Panel D: Steady prognosis, with a median survival of 6 months

The second guide asks you to consider how precise the prognostic statements are. As we mentioned in Section 3a2, investigators study prognosis in a sample of diseased patients, not in the whole population of everyone who has ever had the disease. Purely by the play of chance, then, the identical study done 100 times over with different samples from that same whole population would yield differing results. In deciding whether these prognostic results are important, then, you will need some means of judging just how much these results could vary by chance alone, that is, the precision of the results. This is best done with the 95% confidence interval:* in those 100 repetitions of the identical study with different samples, 95 would be within a calculable distance of the true prognosis (some lower and some higher). For example, an article on the prognosis of first strokes among 675 patients reported a case-fatality rate of 20% in the first month, with the 95% confidence interval of 17–23%; that interval is pretty narrow and if the report was valid, it looks important as well. If, on the other hand, that 20% was based on just 20 patients, the 95% confidence interval on death in the first month would run from 2% to 38% and that is so wide (almost 20-fold) that you couldn't regard the result as important and potentially useful to you. The text, tables or graphs should tell you the confidence interval for the prognosis and you can decide whether it is too big for you to trust it.

That completes your critical appraisal of evidence about prognosis. If you decide that the evidence you've found is both valid and important, you could go to Section 2 of Chapter 4 (page 164) and decide whether and how to apply it to your patient.

* We describe the confidence interval in the Appendix. In this case, the confidence interval on a prognosis (expressed as a decimal) is the observed result plus or minus 1.96 times the square root of {[(the observed result) × (1 – the observed result)] / sample size}. So, for the original study 20% = 0.2 and the confidence interval becomes 0.2 +/– 1.96 times the square root of {[(0.2) × (0.8)]/675} or 0.2 +/– 0.03 or 17–23%. As a check on your understanding, you can see if you can calculate the confidence interval when the sample is just 40 stroke patients.

Further reading

Laupacis A, Wells G, Richardson W S, Tugwell P for the Evidence-Based Medicine Working Group. Users' guides to the medical literature. V. How to use an article about prognosis. JAMA 1994; 272: 234–7.

Section 3b3

Is this evidence about a treatment important?

This section will help you determine the size and potential benefits of the effects of the treatment described in a report, whether you've decided (from the previous section) that the report is valid or whether you start here. Because our primary perspective in this book is the individual clinician, the main measure we will show you how to develop and use is the number of patients a clinician needs to treat in order to prevent one additional adverse outcome (NNT) and along the way we will show you both the absolute risk reduction (ARR) and relative risk reduction (RRR) in the occurrence of adverse outcomes achieved by active therapy. We'll also introduce you to the bare bones of assessing the results of an economic analysis, a more complex method that we employ in determining the effects of therapy when we are taking the broader perspective (usually in collaboration with health managers) of deciding how groups of patients, or society as a whole, should be provided or offered treatments in the way that best uses scarce resources such as hospital beds, drugs, operating time, clinicians and money. Finally, we'll give you a brief description of how evidence on the effects of therapy can be formulated into a clinical decision analysis.

In Section 3 of Chapter 4, we'll show you how to extrapolate the measures from each of these three approaches to individual patients, in order to answer the question: Can I apply these results to my patient?

Is the evidence from this randomized trial important?

Introducing some measures of the effects of therapy

Knowing whether you should be impressed with the results of a valid therapeutic trial requires two steps: first, finding the

most useful clinical expression of these results (or converting data from the report into this most useful expression); and second, comparing those results with the results of other treatments for other conditions. We'll take these one at a time.

The relative risk reduction (RRR)

The Diabetes Control and Complications Trial into the effect of intensive diabetes therapy on the development and progression of neuropathy, which we've summarized in Table 3b3.1, confirmed neuropathy occurred among 9.6% of patients randomized to usual care (1–2 insulin injections/day to prevent glycemic symptoms; we'll call that the control event rate or CER) and 2.8% (we'll call that the experimental event rate or EER) among patients randomized to intensive therapy (insulin pump or =>3 injections per day).

This difference was statistically highly significant, but how might this treatment effect be expressed in terms of its clinical significance? The traditional measure of this effect is the proportional or 'relative' risk reduction (abbreviated RRR in our journal), calculated as (CER–EER)/CER. In this example, the RRR is (9.6% – 2.8%) / 9.6% or 71%; intensive therapy reduced the risk of developing neuropathy by 71%.

Why not confine our description of the clinical significance of this result to the relative risk reduction (RRR)? The reason is that the RRR fails to discriminate huge absolute treatment effects (10 times those observed in this trial) from trivial ones (one ten-thousandth of those observed here). For example, if the rates of neuropathy were 10 times those observed in this trial (the 'high hypothetical case' in Table 3b3.1), and a whopping 96% of control patients and 28% of intensively treated patients developed neuropathy, the relative risk reduction would remain unchanged: RRR = (96% – 28%) / 96% or 71%. And if a trivial 0.00096% of control and 0.00028% of intensively treated patients developed neuropathy (the 'low hypothetical case' in Table 3b3.1), the relative risk reduction is as before: RRR still = (0.00096% − 0.00028%) / 0.00096 = 71%! This is because the relative risk reduction discards the underlying susceptibility (or 'baseline risk') of patients entering randomized trials; as a result, the relative risk reduction cannot discriminate huge risks and benefits from small ones.

The absolute risk reduction (ARR)

In contrast to these non-discriminating relative risk reductions, the absolute difference in the rates of neuropathy between control and experimental patients (CER−EER) clearly does discriminate between these extremes and this measure is called the absolute risk reduction or ARR. In the trial, the ARR or (CER−EER) = 9.6% − 2.8% = 6.8%; in the high hypothetical case, where 96% of control patients and 28% of intensively treated patients developed neuropathy, the ARR = 96% − 28% = 68% and in the low hypothetical case in which a trivial 0.00096% of control and 0.00028% of intensively treated patients developed neuropathy, the ARR = 0.00096% − 0.00028% = 0.00068%. These absolute risk reductions retain the underlying susceptibility of patients and provide more complete information than relative risk reductions. And when treatment increases the occurrence of some good event (rather than decreasing the occurrence of some bad event) we can generate an absolute risk increase or ARI. But, unlike relative risk reductions (RRRs), absolute risk reductions and increases (ARRs and ARIs) are difficult to remember and don't slip easily off the tongue at the bedside (lots of clinicians become queasy with numbers less than 1.0).

The number of patients that need to be treated (NNT) to prevent one bad outcome

If, however, we divide the absolute risk reduction into 1 (that is, if we 'invert' the ARR or 'take its reciprocal' so that it becomes 1/ARR), we generate a very useful number, for it represents the number of patients we need to treat (NNT)

with the experimental therapy in order to prevent one of them from developing the bad outcome.* In this case, we would generate the number of diabetics we would need to treat with the intensive regimen in order to prevent one of them from developing neuropathy. In the trial, the NNT is 1/ARR or 1/6.8% or 14.7; we usually round that number upwards (in this case, to 15) and we now can say that for every 15 patients who are treated with the more intensive insulin regimen, one will be prevented from developing diabetic neuropathy.

Is this a large or a small number of patients that need to be treated to prevent one bad outcome? Now we're ready to pursue that second step in deciding whether to be impressed with the valid results of a therapeutic trial. Like many important matters in medicine, the answer has to do with clinical significance, not statistical significance. This NNT of 15 certainly is far smaller than the number of patients we'd need to treat in the extremely low hypothetical example, in which 1/ARR becomes 1/(0.00068%) or an NNT of more than 147 000, a figure so vast that we can't imagine anyone judging that it was worth the effort. We can get a better idea by comparing this NNT of 15 with that for other interventions we are familiar with in medicine.

In doing so, we add the additional dimension of the duration of therapy: in the diabetes trial treatment went on for an average of 6.5 years, meaning that we need to treat about 15 diabetics for about 6.5 years with an intensive insulin regimen to prevent one of them from developing neuropathy. How does this compare with other treatments, over other durations, for other conditions? We show some of them (with the event rates appearing as decimals rather than percents) in Table 3b3.2. Beginning on an optimistic note, we need to treat only about 20 chest pain patients who appear to be having heart attacks with streptokinase and aspirin to save a life at 5 weeks. On the other hand, we need to treat about 70 elderly hypertensives for 5 years with antihypertensive drugs

---

* Similarly, 1/ARI tells us how many individuals we need to treat to cause one additional good outcome.

Table 3b3.1 Clinically useful measures of the effects of treatment

The occurrence of neuropathy	Event rates (diabetic neuropathy) Usual insulin regimen (CER)	Intensive insulin regimen (EER)	Relative risk reduction RRR = $\dfrac{\text{CER−EER}}{\text{CER}}$	Absolute risk reduction ARR = (CER−EER)	Number needed to be treated (to prevent one event) NNT = 1/ARR
In the actual trial	9.6%	2.8%	$\dfrac{9.6\%-2.8\%}{9.6\%}$ = 71%	9.6%−2.8% = 6.8%	$\dfrac{1}{6.8\%}$ = 14.7 or 15
High hypothetical case A	96%	28%	$\dfrac{96\%-28\%}{96\%}$ = 71%	96%−28% = 68%	$\dfrac{1}{68\%}$ = 1.47 or 2
Low hypothetical case B	0.00096%	0.00028%	$\dfrac{(0.00096\%-0.00028\%)}{0.00096\%}$ = 71%	(0.00096% −0.00028%) = 0.00068%	$\dfrac{1}{0.00068\%}$ = 147 000

to save one life, about 100 men with no evidence of coronary heart disease for 5 years with aspirin to prevent one heart attack and about 10 patients with symptomatic moderate to severe carotid artery stenosis with endarterectomy to prevent one major or fatal stroke over the following 2 years.

We think that the 'number needed to be treated' (NNT) to prevent one event is the most useful measure of the clinical effort we and our patients must expend in order to help them avoid bad outcomes to their illnesses. Note, however, that this is a measure with real meaning for clinicians, but not for individual patients (who are interested in Ns of 1, not NNTs). Furthermore, because we are focusing here on the magnitude of the treatment effect, rather than on the probability that we have drawn a false-positive conclusion that the treatment is at all effective (when it is not), we should employ confidence intervals around the NNT, specifying the 'limits' within which we can confidently state the true NNT lies (95% of the time), rather than focus just on p-values. Readers who want to brush up on confidence intervals can refer to the Appendix.

Since we are interested in the risks as well as the benefits of treatments, we can generate a parallel 'number needed to harm' or NNH to express the downside of therapy. For example, if anticoagulation carries an annual risk of major bleeding of 2%, the NNH is 1/2% = 50.

Overviews and metaanalyses often provide NNTs, but sometimes only report odds ratios. The latter are not the same as RRRs and can be converted into RRRs only when you know the patient's expected event rate (PEER) by using the formula:

$$NNT = \frac{1- [PEER \times (1 - OR)]}{(1 - PEER) \times PEER \times (1 - OR)}$$

To help you 'translate' odds ratios to NNTs (without having to crank through this formula), we've summarized several of them in Table 3b3.3.

The NNT from the published report, in light of your own clinical expertise and compared with those in Table 3b3.2, will give you an idea of whether the treatment is potentially

* Ann Intern Med 1995;122:561-8. EBM 1995;1:9.
† Diabetes Res Clin Pract 1995;28:103-17
‡ Lancet 1988;2:349-60.
§ JAMA 1967;202:116-22.
¶ BMJ 1985;291:97-104.
** N Engl J Med 1995;333:1184-9. EBM 1996;1:87.
†† Lancet 1995;345:1455-63. EBM 1996;1:44.
‡‡ Lancet 1993;341:973-8.
§§ N Engl J Med 1991;325:445-53.
¶¶ Am J Obstet Gynecol 1995;173:322-35. EBM 1996;1:92.

To find more examples, and to nominate additions to the databank of NNTs, refer to this textbook's Web Page at: http://cebm.jr2.ox.ac.uk/

Table 3b3.2 Some NNTs for different treatments

Condition or disorder	Intervention	Events being prevented	Event Rates		Duration of follow-up	NNT to prevent one additional event
			Control Event Rate CER	Experimental Event Rate EER		
Diabetes (IDDM)*	Intensive insulin regimen	Diabetic neuropathy	0.096	0.028	6.5 years	15
Diabetes (NIDDM)†	Intensive insulin regimen	Worse diabetic retinopathy	0.38	0.13	6 years	4
		Nephropathy	0.30	0.10		5
Acute myocardial infarction‡	Streptokinase and Aspirin	Death at 5 weeks	0.134	0.081	5 weeks	19
		Death at 2 years	0.216	0.174	2 years	24
Diastolic blood pressure 115-129 mm Hg§	Antihypertensive drugs	Death, stroke or myocardial infarction	0.1286	0.0137	1.5 years	3
Diastolic blood pressure 90-109 mm Hg¶	Antihypertensive drugs	Death, stroke or myocardial infarction	0.0545	0.0467	5.5 years	128
Independent elderly people**	Comprehensive geriatric home assessment	Long-term nursing home admission	0.10	0.04	3 years	17
Pregnant woman with eclampsia††	iv MgSO4 (vs. diazepam)	Recurrent convulsion	0.279	0.132	hours	7
Healthy women ages 50-69‡‡	Breast examination plus mammography	Death from breast cancer	0.00345	0.00252	9 years	1075
Symptomatic high-grade carotid artery stenosis§§	Carotid endarterectomy	Major stroke or death	0.181	0.08	2 years	10
Preterm babies¶¶	Antenatal corticosteroids	Respiratory distress syndrome	0.23	0.13	days	11

Table 3b3.3 Translating odds ratios to NNTs

	Odds ratio				
	0.9	0.8	0.7	0.6	0.5
Patient's expected event rate (PEER)					
.05	209*	104	69	52	41†
.10	110	54	36	27	21
.20	61	30	20	14	11
.30	46	22	14	10	8
.40	40	19	12	9	7
.50	38	18	11	8	6
.70	44	20	13	9	6
.90	101‡	46	27	18	12§

The numbers in the body of the table are the NNTs for the corresponding odds ratios at that particular patient's expected event rate (PEER).
* The relative risk reduction (RRR) here is 10%.
† The RRR here is 49%.
‡ The RRR here is 1%.
§ The RRR here is 9%.

useful for your patient. In the next chapter, we will show you a very simple way to find out whether this potential is met for your individual patient.

Section 3b4

Is this evidence about harm important?

The main measure that indicates whether valid evidence that a treatment harms some patients is also impressive (and potentially useful clinically) is the strength of the association between receiving the treatment and suffering the adverse effect. Strength here means the risk or odds of the adverse effect with, as opposed to without, exposure to the treatment; the higher the risk or odds, the greater the strength and the more you should be impressed with it.

Different tactics for estimating the strength of association are used in different types of studies and these are shown in Table 3b4.1. In the randomized trial and cohort study, patients who were and were not exposed to the treatment are carefully followed up to find out whether they develop the adverse outcome, with the risk in the treated patients, rela-

Table 3b4.1 Different ways of calculating the strength of an association between a treatment and subsequent adverse outcomes

		Adverse outcome		Totals
		Present (Case)	Absent (Control)	
Exposed to the treatment	Yes (Cohort)	a	b	a+b
	No (Cohort)	c	d	c+d
	Totals	a+c	b+d	a+b+c+d

In a randomized trial or cohort study: relative risk = RR = [a/(a+b)]/[c/(c+d)]
In a case-control study: relative odds = RO = **ad/bc**

tive to untreated patients, calculated as [a/(a+b)]/[c/(c+d)]. Thus, if 1000 patients receive a treatment and 20 of them have an adverse outcome, **a**=20 and **a/(a+b)** = 20/1000 = 2%; and if just two of 1000 patients with the same condition but receiving a different treatment suffered this adverse outcome, **c**=2 and **c/(c+d)** = 2/1000 = 0.2% and the relative risk = 2%/0.2% or 10. That is, patients receiving the suspect treatment were 10 times as likely to suffer the adverse outcome as patients treated some other way.

In a case-control study, where patients with and without the adverse outcome are selected and tracked backward to their prior treatments, strength (which in this case is called the odds ratio) can only be indirectly estimated as **ad/bc**. For example, if 100 cases of the adverse outcome are assembled and it is discovered that 90 of them had received the suspect treatment, **a**=90 and **c**=10; if 100 control patients, free of the adverse outcome, are also assembled and it is discovered that only 45 of them received the suspect treatment, **b**=45 and **d**=55, and the relative odds = **ad/bc** = (90×55)/(45×10) = 11. That is, patients receiving the suspect treatment are 11 times as likely to suffer the adverse event as patients treated some other way.

How big should relative risks and relative odds become before you should be impressed with them? This question has two answers. First, you'd like to be confident that the relative risk (RR) or relative odds (RO) is really greater than 1 (when RR or RO = 1, the adverse outcome is no greater with than without exposure to the suspect treatment). So, as before, you'd want to be sure that the entire confidence interval remains within a clinically important range of RR or RO. Second, the size of the 'impressive' RR or RO depends on the type of study from which it is generated. Because of the biases we described in case-control studies, you'd want to be sure that the RO was greater than that which could arise from bias alone and you might not want to become impressed with their ROs until they reach 4 or more (some of our colleagues would relax these guides for a serious adverse effect and set them even higher for a trivial one). Since cohort studies are less subject to bias, you might be impressed with RRs of 3 or

Table 4.1.1 Questions to answer in applying a valid diagnostic test to an individual patient

1. Is the diagnostic test available, affordable, accurate and precise in your setting?
2. Can you generate a clinically sensible estimate of your patient's pretest probability:
   - from practice data?
   - from personal experience?
   - from the report itself?
   - from clinical speculation?
3. Will the resulting post-test probabilities affect your management and help your patient?
   - Could it move you across a test–treatment threshold?
   - Would your patient be a willing partner in carrying it out?
   - Would the consequences of the test help your patient reach their goals in all this?

Section 4.1

Can you apply this valid, important evidence about a diagnostic test in caring for your patient?

Having found a valid systematic review or individual report about a diagnostic test and decided that its accuracy is sufficiently high to be useful, how do you integrate it with your individual clinical expertise and apply it to your patient?

There are three questions whose answers dictate this determination, summarized in Table 4.1.1. First, is the diagnostic test available, affordable, accurate and precise in your setting? You obviously can't order a test that's not available but even if it is, you may want to check around to be sure that it's performed and interpreted in a competent, reproducible fashion and that its potential consequences (see below) justify its cost. Moreover, diagnostic tests often behave differently among different subsets of patients, generating higher likelihood ratios in later stages of florid disease and lower likelihood ratios in early, mild stages. This is another reason why multilevel likelihood ratios are helpful, as there are at least theoretical reasons why they should suffer less distortion from this cause. Finally, it is known that at least some diagnostic tests based on symptoms or signs lose power as patients move from primary care to secondary and tertiary care. Reference back to Table 3b1.1 can show you why: if patients are referred onward in part because of symptoms, their primary care clinicians will be sending along patients in both cells a and b and subsequent evaluations of the accuracy of their symptoms will tend to show falling specificity due to the referral of patients with false-positive findings. If you think that any of these factors may be operating, you can try out what you judge to be clinically sensible variations in the likelihood ratios for your test result and see whether the results alter your post-test probabilities in a way that changes your diagnosis (the short-hand term for this sort of exploration is 'sensitivity analysis').

The second question you need to answer is whether you can generate a clinically sensible estimate of your patient's pretest probability. Sometimes you've actually got the data on pretest probabilities from your practice or institution. That's wonderful when it exists and constitutes a reason to consider keeping some records on the pretest probabilities for important diagnoses you eventually make for the specific presenting complaints in which you'd consider this sort of diagnostic test. Sometimes, you've had enough experience both to be able to make this estimation based on your own experience and to know how your estimate can be distorted by your last case (either way, depending on whether you ruled in or ruled out the diagnosis), your most dramatic or embarrassing case (usually this either distorts your pretest odds upwards or makes you reluctant to quit testing until the post-test odds are vanishingly small) or by whether you are an expert in the evaluation or care of patients with this diagnosis (which usually makes you reluctant to miss one).

Early in your career or when you haven't previously encountered this diagnostic situation, you'll be less certain about your patient's pretest probability. When that happens, you can try one or more of the following. First, if

more in them. And because randomized trials are relatively free of bias, any RR whose confidence interval excludes 1 is impressive and warrants further consideration.

Having decided that you are impressed with both the validity and the strength of the relationship between the suspect treatment and the adverse outcome, you then need to translate this into some measure of the impact of changing your treatment strategy on the occurrence of the adverse outcome and decide whether it is worth the effort required to achieve it. The measures we've employed up to now, the RR and OR, don't provide this information very well and you need to return to the concept of the NNT. In this case you are concerned about a bad outcome and you might want to revise the term to the 'number of patients needed to be treated to produce one episode of harm' or NNH. Our reason for doing this is that the RR and OR are fine for determining whether the link to harm was true, but don't tell us whether the link was clinically important. For example, a cohort study showed that NSAIDS can cause gastrointestinal bleeding and the confidence interval on the relative risk for this adverse outcome included 2. A randomized trial showed that the antiarrhythmic drugs encainide and flecainide can cause death and the confidence interval on the relative risk for this adverse outcome also included 2. But the absolute increase in the risk of bleeding in the former study was small, at about 0.05%, which translates to an NNH of 2000 to cause one more GI bleed, whereas the absolute increase in the risk of death in the latter trial was 4.7% or an NNH of 21 to cause one additional death! Clearly, similar RRs or ORs can lead to very different NNHs and you need the latter as well as the former to make your clinical decision about your patient.

That final step of integrating this external evidence with your clinical expertise is discussed in Section 4.4.

Further reading

Levine M, Walter S D, Lee H, Haines T, Holbrook A, Moyer V for the Evidence-Based Medicine Working Group. Users' guides to the medical literature. IV. How to use an article about harm. JAMA 1994; 271: 1615–19.

your setting and patient closely resemble those that appeared in the report, you can use its pretest probability. Or if your patient is a bit different from those in the study, you can use its pretest probability as a starting point and again set off on a sensitivity analysis using clinically sensible variations in pretest probabilities and determining their impact on the test's usefulness. As before, the issue here is not whether your patient is exactly like those in the report, but whether they are so different that the report is of no help in making the diagnosis. Finally, you may simply go straight to a sensitivity analysis in which you plug the likelihood ratios from your report into a range of sensible pretest probabilities and see what the likely range of post-test probabilities will be (perhaps using the entries in Table 3b1.4 on page 124 to help you).

The final question you need to answer is: Will the resulting post-test probabilities affect your management and help your patient? The elements of this answer are three. First, could its results move you across some threshold that would cause you to stop all further testing? Two thresholds should be borne in mind. If the diagnostic test was negative or generated a likelihood ratio well below 1.0, the post-test probability might become so low that you would abandon the diagnosis it was pursuing and turn to other diagnostic possibilities. Put in terms of thresholds, this negative test result has moved you from above to below the 'test threshold' and you won't do any more tests for that diagnostic possibility. On the other hand, if the diagnostic test came back positive or generated a high likelihood ratio, the post-test probability might become so high that you would also abandon further testing because you'd made your diagnosis and would now move to choosing the most appropriate therapy; in these terms, you've now crossed from below to above the 'treatment threshold'. It's only if your diagnostic test result leaves you stranded between the test and treatment thresholds that you'd continue to pursue that initial diagnosis by performing other tests. Although there are some very fancy ways of calculating test and treatment thresholds from test accuracy and the risks and benefits of correct and incorrect

diagnostic conclusions,* intuitive test–treatment thresholds are commonly used by experienced clinicians and are another example of individual clinical expertise.

You may not cross a test–treatment threshold until you've performed several different diagnostic tests and here is where another nice property of the likelihood ratio comes into play. Because the post-test odds for the first diagnostic test you apply are the pretest odds for your second diagnostic test, you needn't switch back and forth between odds and probabilities between tests. You can simply keep multiplying the running product by the likelihood ratio generated from the next test. For example, when a 45-year-old man walks into your office his pretest probability of $\geq 75\%$ stenosis of one or more of his coronary arteries is about 6%. Suppose that he gives you a history of atypical chest pain (only two of the three symptoms of substernal chest discomfort, brought on by exertion, and relieved in <10 minutes by rest: a likelihood ratio of about 13) and that his exercise ECG reveals 2.2 mm of non-sloping ST-segment depression (a likelihood ratio of about 11). Then his post-test probability for coronary stenosis is his pretest probability [converted into odds] times the product of the likelihood ratios generated from his history (13) and exercise ECG (11), with the resulting post-test odds converted back to probabilities (through dividing by its value + 1): $(0.06 / 0.94) \times 13 \times 11 = 9.13 / 10.13 = 90\%$. The final result of these calculations is strictly accurate as long as the diagnostic tests being combined are 'independent' (that is, the probability of a specific result on the second is the same for any result on the first) and we know intuitively that this is not true for most of the diagnostic tests we apply in sequences aiming toward a single diagnosis. Accordingly, we'd want the calculated post-test probability at the end of this sequence to be comfortably above our treatment threshold before we would act upon it. This additional example of how likelihood ratios make lots of implicit diagnostic reasoning explicit is another argument in favor of generating overall

---

* See the recommendations for further reading or N Engl J Med 1980; 302: 1109.

likelihood ratios for sequences or clusters of diagnostic tests, as suggested back in Section 3b1.

We hope that you involved your patient as you worked your way through all the foregoing considerations that lead you to think that the diagnostic test is worth considering. If you haven't, you certainly need to do so now. Every diagnostic test involves some invasion of privacy and some are embarrassing, painful or dangerous. You'll have to be sure that the patient is an informed, willing partner in the undertaking.

Finally, the ultimate question to ask about using any diagnostic test is whether its consequences (reassurance when negative, labeling and possibly generating awful diagnostic and prognostic news if positive, leading to further diagnostic tests and treatments, etc.) will help your patient achieve their goals of therapy. Included here are considerations of how subsequent interventions match clinical guidelines or restrictions on access to therapy designed to optimize the use of finite resources for all members of your society.

Further reading

Jaeschke R, Guyatt G H, Sackett D L for the Evidence-Based Medicine Working Group. Users' guides to the medical literature. VI. How to use an article about a diagnostic test. B. What are the results and will they help me in caring for my patients? JAMA 1994; 271: 703–7.

Section 4.2

Can you apply this valid, important evidence about prognosis in caring for your patient?

Having decided that the evidence you tracked down about prognosis is both valid and important, you now can consider how to use it in your clinical practice. Two guides can help you make these judgments; they appear in Table 4.2.1 and will be considered here.

First, were the study patients sufficiently similar to your own? The first guide asks you to compare your patients to those in the article and since presumably you know your patients well, this means trying to get to know the study patients well enough to compare them. Look for descriptions of the study sample, including the patients' demographics and important clinical characteristics. The more the study patients are like your patients, the more readily you can apply the results to your patients. Inevitably, some differences will turn up, so how similar is similar enough? To help you with this judgment, as in other places in this book, we suggest that you try this question framed the other way: are the study patients so different from yours that you'd expect their outcomes to be so different that they wouldn't be any use to you in making prognostic predictions about your patients?

Second, will this evidence make a clinically important impact on your conclusions about what to offer or tell your patient? If the evidence suggests a good prognosis when patients (especially in the early stages of disease) remain

Table 4.2.1 Can you apply this valid, important evidence about prognosis in caring for your patient?

1. Were the study patients similar to your own?
2. Will this evidence make a clinically important impact on your conclusions about what to offer or tell your patient?

untreated, that could strongly influence your discussion of treatment options with them. If, on the other hand, prognostic information derived from a control group in a randomized trial suggests a gloomy prognosis when no definitive therapy is instituted, your message to your patient would reflect this fact. And even when the prognostic evidence doesn't lead to a treat/don't treat decision, valid evidence is always useful in providing your patient or their family with the information they want to have about what the future is likely to hold for them and their illness.

Further reading

Laupacis A, Wells G, Richardson W S, Tugwell P for the Evidence-Based Medicine Working Group. Users' guides to the medical literature. V. How to use an article about prognosis. JAMA 1994; 272: 234–7.

Section 4.3

Can you apply this valid, important evidence about a treatment in caring for your patient?

In deciding whether valid, potentially useful results apply to your patient, you need once again to integrate the evidence with your clinical expertise. As shown in Table 4.3.1, there are two elements to this integration. The first estimates the impact of the treatment on patients just like yours and the second compares the values and preferences of your patient with the regimen and its consequences.

Estimating the impact of a valid, important treatment result on an individual patient

This element poses two additional questions: Do these results apply to your patient? How great would the potential benefit of therapy actually be for your individual patient?

Do these results apply to your patient?

Your patient wasn't in the trial that established the efficacy of this treatment. Maybe (because of their age, sex, comorbidity, disease severity or for a host of other sociodemographic, biologic or clinical reasons) they wouldn't even have been eligible for the trial. How can you extrapolate* from the external evidence to your individual patient? Rather than slavishly asking: 'Would my patient satisfy the eligibility criteria for the trial?' and rejecting its usefulness if they didn't exactly fit every one of them, we'd suggest bringing in some of your knowledge of human biology and

---

* Some teachers call this 'generalizing' from the trial, but really it's 'particularizing' to an individual patient, not generalizing to all patients, everywhere. Accordingly, we'll use the more generic term 'extrapolating'.

Table 4.3.1 Are these valid, potentially useful results applicable to your patient?

1. Do these results apply to your patient?
   - Is your patient so different from those in the trial that its results can't help you?
   - How great would the potential benefit of therapy actually be for your individual patient?
2. Are your patient's values and preferences satisfied by the regimen and its consequences?
   - Do your patient and you have a clear assessment of their values and preferences?
   - Are they met by this regimen and its consequences?

clinical experience, turning the question around and asking: 'Is my patient so different from those in the trial that its results cannot help me make my treatment decision?' Pharmacogenetics aside, there are very few situations in which you would expect a drug or diet or operation to produce qualitatively different results in patients inside a trial and those who don't quite fit its eligibility criteria. Only if you conclude that your patient is so different from those in the study that its results simply don't inform your treatment decision should you discard its results.

What about subgroups?

Sometimes treatments appear to benefit some subgroups of patients but not others. For example, some of the early trials of aspirin for transient ischemic attacks suggested that this drug was efficacious in men but not in women. As is usually the case, this 'qualitative' difference in the effects of therapy (helpful for one group but useless or harmful in another) was a chance finding and later trials and overviews confirmed that aspirin is efficacious in women. The results from megatrials and overviews suggest that extrapolations from the overall results of individual trials usually are correct when applied to subgroups of patients in those trials. If you think that you may be dealing with one of the exceptions to this rule and that the treatment you're examining really does work in a qualitatively different way among

Table 4.3.2 Should you believe apparent qualitative differences in the efficacy of therapy in some subgroups of patients?

Only if you can say 'yes' to all of the following:
1. Does it really make biologic and clinical sense?
2. Is the qualitative difference both clinically (beneficial for some but useless or harmful for others) and statistically significant?
3. Was it hypothesized before the study began (rather than the product of dredging the data) and has it been confirmed in other, independent studies?
4. Was it one of just a few subgroup analyses carried out in this study?

different patients, you should apply the guides in Table 4.3.2. In particular, unless this difference in response makes biologic sense, was hypothesized before the trial and has been confirmed in a second, independent trial, we'd suggest that you accept the treatment's overall efficacy as the best estimate of its efficacy in your patient.

So, unless there is some really powerful biologic reason for you to think that the treatment, if accepted by your patient, would be totally ineffectual or act in the opposing direction from the way it acted in patients in the study, we think you have good grounds for extrapolating the direction of the effect of the treatment on your patient's illness. Having decided that the direction of the treatment effect is likely to be the same as that observed in the study, you can now turn to considering whether that effect is likely to be great or small.

How great would the potential benefit of therapy be for your individual patient?

The trial report informed you about how the treatment worked in the average patient in the trial. How can you translate this to the probable treatment effect in your individual patient? We suggest that the measure we used to decide whether the treatment was potentially useful, the number of patients you need to treat (NNT) to prevent one bad outcome, is useful here. The trick is to translate the NNT

from the study into an NNT that fits your patient. You can do this the longer, harder (and maybe more accurate*) way or the quick and easy (but maybe less accurate) way.

The long way is to estimate the absolute susceptibility of your individual patient for developing the bad outcome over a period of time equal to the duration of the study. If the study you're using had a placebo or no-treatment group or subgroup with features like your patient, you could use their susceptibility† for this purpose. Another way would be to carry out a literature search to find a paper on the prognosis of patients like yours and use that figure. Either way, you'd take the resulting susceptibility (you could express it as a decimal fraction or a percentage, whichever you're more comfortable using) and multiply it by the RRR from the study. The result is the ARR and you can invert it to get the NNT. For example, if you find a prognosis paper suggesting that the susceptibility of your patient for a bad outcome is about 0.4 (the term we use to describe that susceptibility is the 'patient expected event rate' or PEER, so PEER = 40%) over a period of time equal to the duration of the trial that generated an RRR of 50%. Assuming that this RRR applies regardless of the susceptibility of patients in that trial, the ARR is PEER × RRR = 40% × 50% = 20% and the corresponding NNT is 1/ARR = 1/20% = 5 and you'd need to treat just five patients like yours for that length of time to prevent one event. If you would like to avoid these calculations, you can use the nomogram that appears in Figure 4.3.1. But there is an even easier way to estimate an NNT for patients like yours.

As we stated in the previous chapter, one of the reasons why the NNT is useful when interpreting the results of treatment trials is the ease with which it can be extrapolated to your own practice and to individual patients outside the trials. Through some very simple arithmetic, you can estimate NNTs for specific patients. All you need do is estimate the

* We're not being cute here. We all are pretty new at this and really don't know!
† Some people, especially when they use a control group to estimate susceptibility, call it 'baseline risk'.

susceptibility of your individual patient (if they were to receive just the control treatment) relative to the average control patient in the reported trial and convert this estimate into a decimal fraction we'll call F (if you judge your patient to be twice as susceptible as those in the trial, F = 2; if your patient is only half as susceptible as the average control patient in the trial, F = 0.5, and if just like the patients in the trial, F = 1). As long as the treatment produces a constant relative risk reduction across the spectrum of susceptibilities,* the NNT for your patient is simply the reported NNT divided by F. Going back to our intensive insulin example in Section 3b3, we learned that a group of clinical investigators had to treat 15 diabetics with intensive insulin regimens for 6.5 years in order to prevent one of them from developing diabetic neuropathy (NNT=15). If you judge that your patient was only half as susceptible as patients in that trial, F = 0.5 and NNT/F = 15/0.5 = 30, so 30 of these less susceptible patients would need to be treated for about 6.5 years with the intensive insulin regimen to prevent one of them from going on to develop neuropathy.

Comparing the values and preferences of your patient with the regimen and its consequences

A return to Table 4.3.1 identifies the steps to be taken here. You and your patient need to achieve a clear assessment of their values and preferences and then determine whether they will be served by the regimen in question. Sometimes the answer will be evident in a few seconds: for a patient having a heart attack, the value of survival and the preference for a simple, low-risk intervention like aspirin, given the efficacy of this regimen, usually makes this decision quickly agreed and acted upon. Other times the answer will take weeks and several visits to sort out: radiation or

* This is a big assumption and we're only beginning to learn when assuming a constant RRR is appropriate (for lots of medical treatments like antihypertensive drugs) and inappropriate (for some operations like carotid endarterectomy, where the RRR rises with increasing susceptibility).

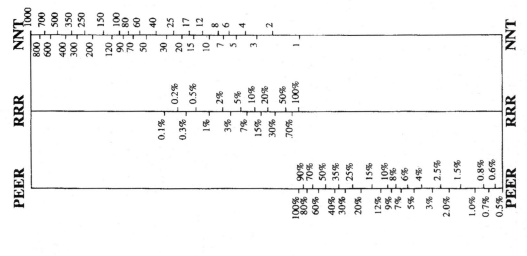

PEER	RRR	NNT
100%		1000 — 800
80%		700 — 600
60%		500 — 400
50%		350 — 300
40%		250 — 200
35%		150 — 120
30%	0.1%	100 — 90
25%	0.2% — 0.3%	80 — 70
20%	0.5%	60 — 50
15%	1%	40 — 30
12%	2%	25 — 20
10%	3%	17 — 15
9%	5%	12 — 10
8%	7%	8 — 7
7%	10%	6 — 5
6%	15%	4 — 3
5%	20%	
4%	30%	2
3%	50%	
2.5%	70%	
2.0%	100%	1
1.5%		
1.0%		
0.8%		
0.7%		
0.6%		
0.5%		
PEER	**RRR**	**NNT**

Figure 4.3.1 A nomogram for determining NNTs. Reprinted with permission from Chatellier G et al. The number needed to treat: a clinically useful nomogram in its proper context. BMJ 1996; 312: 426–9.

adjuvant chemotherapy for stage II carcinoma of the breast or transurethral resection of the prostate for moderate symptoms of prostatism.

Section 4.4

Can you apply this valid, important evidence about harm in caring for your patient?

In deciding whether and how to apply valid, potentially important results of a critical appraisal about a harmful treatment to an individual patient, four aspects of individual clinical expertise are important and they are listed in Table 4.4.1.

First, you need to decide whether the results of your critical appraisal can be extrapolated to your patient. As before, the issue is not whether your patient would have met all the inclusion criteria for the systematic review or individual study that demonstrated the harmful effect of the treatment, but whether your patient is so different from those in the report that its results provide no useful guidance for you.

Second, you need to estimate your patient's risk of the adverse outcome relative to the patients in the report. As we described in Section 4.3, if you can express this as a decimal fraction we'll call F (if your patient is twice the risk of those in the report, F=2; if half the risk, F=0.5; if the same risk, F=1) you can then simply divide the number of patients needed to be treated to produce one episode of harm (NNH) from the report by F. If, for example, you decided that a patient you're considering placing on an NSAID is at four times the risk of an upper GI bleed as those in a cohort study

Table 4.4.1 Should these valid, potentially important results of a critical appraisal about a harmful drug change the treatment of an individual patient?

1. Can the study results be extrapolated to this patient?
2. What are this patient's risks of the adverse outcome?
3. What are this patient's preferences, concerns and expectations from this treatment?
4. What alternative treatments are available?

---

that generated an NNH of 2000, the appropriate NNH for your patient becomes 2000/4 = 500.

Third, as with all clinical decisions, you need to identify and incorporate your patient's preferences, concerns and expectations into your recommendation. If they are 'risk-averse', on the one hand, or willing to gamble side-effects to gain possible treatment benefit, on the other, your discussions of the risks and benefits of the same treatment, even among patients with identical NNHs, may lead to very different treatment plans. At this point you can further modify NNH (or its F, whichever you are more comfortable dealing with) to take into account both your own and your patient's thoughts about the comparative health impacts of the treatment's adverse effect and the clinical event it was being used to prevent in the first place (represented by its NNT). If your patient is risk averse or if either of you thinks that the treatment's adverse effect (e.g. an intracranial bleed from anti-coagulants) is 2–3 times as severe as the event the treatment was intended to prevent (recurrent deep vein thrombosis), you could double or triple the F for the NNH (or cut the NNH by 1/2 or 2/3) and then see how it compares with the NNT. If, on the other hand, your patient is a risk taker or the adverse treatment effect (e.g. cough from an ACE inhibitor) was only 1% as severe as the event the treatment was intended to prevent (death from heart failure), you could reduce the F for the NNH to 0.01 or multiply the NNH by 100.* In either case, the comparison of the treatment's 'adjusted' NNH with its NNT becomes very informative. If a treatment's NNH, after all this adjustment, is lower than its NNT, shouldn't you be considering some therapeutic alternatives? If your time and resources permit, this would be an ideal situation in which to carry out a clinical decision analysis.

Even if the adjusted NNH exceeds the NNT, you still ought to identify the possible alternative treatments (including no treatment!) you could offer your patient instead of the one

---

* In similar fashion, when a treatment (e.g. NSAIDs for arthritis) causes multiple adverse effects, you would apply a smaller F (or higher NNH) for a minor one (e.g. indigestion) than a major one (e.g. GI hemorrhage).

---

that produces this adverse effect. If a patient experienced wheezing when their hypertension was treated with a beta-blocker, it is easy to substitute another antihypertensive drug that is free of this side-effect. On the other hand, the alternatives to oral contraceptives for temporary conception control may not be acceptable to your patient, despite the small but real risk of thromboembolism from these drugs.

Further reading

Levine M. Walter S D. Lee H, Haines T, Holbrook A, Moyer V for the Evidence-Based Medicine Working Group. Users' guides to the medical literature. IV. How to use an article about harm. JAMA 1994; 271: 1615–19.

Section 4.6

Teaching methods relevant to the clinical application of the results of critical appraisals to individual patients

In this section we will present some strategies and tactics for teaching learners how to apply the results of their critical appraisals to patients. Because EBM begins and ends with patients, it is natural for us to use patient encounters for closing this loop. The message here is that critical appraisal and other elements of EBM are integral components of the everyday bedside and other clinical discussions of how to diagnose and manage patients and not peripheral topics to be discussed at other places and only when time permits. We will start with some obvious clinical situations, but then move progressively farther afield to demonstrate that closely similar strategies and tactics can be applied to a wide variety of teaching and learning situations. Finally, we will describe how several centers and academic consortia around the world operate 5-day workshops on how to practice EBM.

Working rounds on individual patients

First we will consider the 'working round' in which a clinical team review the problems and progress of patients on a clinical service or in an outpatient setting. These are held in various formats. On an inpatient unit, they might consist of a walking round in which every patient on the service is briefly presented, seen and discussed. In an outpatient setting, they might focus on a single patient who has been asked to stay behind or might consider the entire session's patients after they've left. Finally, they might be quite informal gatherings over coffee in which discussions around patients are tagged onto meetings that deal largely with administrative and housekeeping tasks. When the available time is in harmony with the numbers of patients to be seen

(or at least discussed), these can provide excellent opportunities for teaching and learning EBM. Often, however, time is short and the list of patients long and in those circumstances many services adopt a two-stage approach in which they begin by sitting down and quickly reviewing the patient list and then focus on just those patients in whom major decisions have to be made. In either format, patients are presented (and, if available, examined), followed by discussions in which management decisions are taken and defended with the best available evidence. How might these discussions be organized to maximize the opportunities for learning and practicing EBM? Two tactics are useful here.

The first ties EBM to the presentation of the patient. Back in Chapter 1 we described how the educational prescription could be used to initiate finding and critically appraising evidence and in Table 1.5 we showed how it could form the final element in presenting a new patient. In a similar fashion, as shown in Table 4.6.1, filling that educational Rx can form the final element of presenting a patient already known to the clinical service. In this fashion, the scientific justification for a diagnostic or therapeutic course of action becomes part of describing the past and planning the future care of the patient and serves the decision-making as well as educational requirements of the meeting.

The second tactic concerns the actual presentation of the evidence. The busier the service, the more important that evidence central to management decisions is concisely and quickly presented. This is where the CATs (introduced back in Section 3b7) can come in so handy.* After hearing about and (if possible) examining the patient, the team can gather around the resulting CAT, quickly decide whether its clinical bottom line applies, make the management decision and get on to the next patient (requesting copies of CATs for further study or later use).

* For greatest effect, CATs have to be produced in real time while decisions are being made (often easier between visits in ambulatory settings than overnight in inpatient settings). To speed their production, a CAT-Maker is available on disk or via the Website at the Oxford Centre for Evidence-Based Medicine (http://cebm.jr2.ox.ac.uk/).

Table 4.6.1 A guide for learners in presenting an 'OLD'* patient at follow-up rounds

The presentation should summarize 20 things in less than 2 minutes:

1. The patient's surname.
2. Their age.
3. Their gender.
4. Their occupation/social role.
5. When they were admitted.
6. Their chief complaint(s) that led directly to their admission.
7. The number of ACTIVE PROBLEMS that they have at the present time.

And then, for each ACTIVE PROBLEM (a problem could be a symptom, sign, event, diagnosis, injury, psychological state, social predicament, etc.):

8. Its most important symptoms, if any.
9. Its most important signs, if any.
10. The results of diagnostic or other exploratory/confirmatory investigations.
11. The explanation (diagnosis or state) for the problem.
12. The treatment plan instituted for the problem.
13. The response to this treatment plan.
14. The future plans for managing this problem.

Repeat 8–14 for each ACTIVE PROBLEM.

15. Your plans for discharge, posthospital care and follow-up.
16. Whether you've filled the educational prescription that you requested when this patient was admitted (in order to better understand the patient's pathophysiology, clinical findings, diagnosis, prognosis, therapy, prevention of recurrence, quality of care or other important issue in order to become a better clinician).

If so:

17. How you found the relevant evidence.
18. What you found. The clinical bottom line derived from that evidence.
19. Your critical appraisal of that evidence for its VALIDITY and APPLICABILITY.
20. How that critically appraised evidence will alter your care of that (or the next similar) patient

If not, when you are going to fill it.

---

* That is, a patient already known to the service.

The sorts of words you might use:
A. Mr/Mrs/Ms/Prof/PC 11111 is a 22222 year-old 33333 44444 who was admitted on 55555 with the chief complaint of 66666.
B. They have 77777 Active Problems.
C. The first active problem is
   It is characterized by 88888 and 99999 and we
   performed a   which revealed 10-10-10-10.
   We decided that the cause for this problem was
   11-11-11-11 and we started 12-12-12-12 to which
   he/she responded with 13-13-13-13. We plan to
   14-14-14-14.
D. The second/third/fourth active problem is
   (repeat 8-14)
E. At the time of her/his admission, I didn't understand
        as well as I'd like to and I requested
   an educational Rx to answer the question:

I found the relevant evidence by 17-17-17-17 and its clinical bottom line is 18-18-18-18. I believe that this bottom line is/is not valid because 19a-19a-19a-19a and I believe that it is/is not applicable because 19b-19b-19b-19b. I therefore plan to manage this and future, similar patients by 20-20-20-20.

Small groups and 'academic half-days'

Quite often, learners from different clinical teams gather at regularly scheduled educational sessions to receive general instruction in the evaluation and management of patients. The numbers of learners at these sessions can range from a handful to a half-full and running them on a 'set-piece' lecture format can tax the ability of the teachers to stay enthused and the ability of the learners to stay awake. An alternative approach builds on the self-directed, problem-based EBM learning orientation and runs as follows:

1. Learners are asked to identify clinical problems for which they are uncertain about the best way to diagnose or manage affected patients (stating their uncertainties in the form of clinical questions, as in Chapter 1, specifying the patient, the intervention and the outcome of interest to them). Training programs employing this approach report a distinct pattern in the problems that learners identify. Early on, post-graduates identify medical emergencies in which they are unsure of their skills at diagnosing and managing life-threatening situations. Many programs anticipate these concerns and have basic and advanced cardiac and/or trauma support training at the ready.

2. Once the foregoing concerns are addressed, postgraduates identify a wide array of management problems in which they are not sure how to treat patients with specific disorders, followed by clinical problems in diagnosis, prognosis and etiology (especially for iatrogenic disorders). Occasionally, interest is expressed in a locally occurring quality of care study or audit, in their own continuing education, and in health economics. When several learners identify the same clinical situation,* it joins the schedule for a future session and the following processes occur:

● Acting in rotation, one or more of the learners takes on the task of searching the clinical literature for valid, relevant systematic reviews or primary articles on the clinical problem. Along the way, with help from librarians as needed, they develop and hone their skills in searching for the best evidence.

● With faculty guidance, they pick the one or two articles of highest validity and relevance and these, along with a description of the clinical problem, are copied and distributed to everyone to be studied in advance of the session.

● At that session, and again with faculty guidance as needed, they lead the discussion of the validity and potential usefulness of the evidence presented in the paper. Presenters often aid the discussion by introducing CATs or other summaries and displays of the most relevant evidence. This critical appraisal is integrated with discussions of the related pathophysiology and clinical skills, with the final objective of generating a common, evidence-based approach to the clinical

* Part of an initial session can be devoted to reaching consensus on priority clinical problems and such discussions can be repeated as current topics are exhausted and new topics arise.

problem. In some cases, the learners may want to work with senior clinicians to generate and circulate their own guidelines for future use.

Over the years, teachers of EBM have discovered lots of ways *not* to teach effectively and several ways that seem to work. We have summarized them in the form of a set of teaching tips, which appear in Table 4.6.2.

Journal clubs

Journal clubs are dying or dead in many clinical centers, especially when they rely on a rota through which members are asked to summarize the latest issues of preassigned journals. When you think about it, that sort of journal club is run by the postman, not the clinicians or patients, and it is no wonder that it is becoming extinct. On the other hand, a few journal clubs are flourishing and a growing number of them are designed and conducted along EBM lines. They operate like the 'academic half-days' described above.

Each meeting of the journal club has three parts:

1. In one part, journal club members describe patients who exemplify clinical situations which they are uncertain how best to diagnose or manage. This discussion continues until there is consensus that a particular clinical problem,* which we'll call problem C, is worth the time and effort necessary to find its solution. Then either the member who nominated the problem or another member, based on a rota, takes responsibility for performing a search for the best evidence on problem C.

2. In a second part, the results of the evidence search on last session's problem (we'll call it problem B) are shared in the form of photocopies of the abstracts of 4–6 systematic reviews, original articles or other evidence. Club members decide which one or two pieces of evidence are worth studying and arrangements are made to get copies of the clinical problem statement and best evidence to all members well in advance of the next meeting.

* Stated (as in Chapter 1) in terms of a patient, an intervention (and a comparison intervention if appropriate) and an outcome.

Table 4.6.2 Some teaching tips for EBM*

Motivating learning

A. Keep the session relevant and meaningful to learners.

1. Select (or help them track down) articles that relate to patients in their care and pick 'good' articles. Types of good articles for critical appraisal purposes (in decreasing order of their liveliness potential) include those that provide:
   - ground-breaking but solid evidence at the forefront of clinical practice (especially if not yet in widespread use);
   - solid evidence that a common practice is worthless;
   - solid evidence that a common practice ought to be questioned;
   - for common or controversial practices:
     (i) a pair of articles – a bad one to trash, maybe after reading no further than the methods, plus a good one to use for decision making or,
     (ii) a bad article with high trash titres but nonetheless the best one available;
   - NOTE: solid evidence supporting current practice is an excellent place to start (so as to avoid cynicism or nihilism) but risks boring more experienced learners.

2. Start sessions with a patient's problem (real or simulated) and end sessions by coming to a conclusion about how to manage the patient

3. Save time for closure. Come to closure about both the article and the patient. Closure does not necessarily require unanimous agreement. The group may agree that the evidence is fairly solid but still not agree on individuals' decisions for the patient in the scenario.

4. If a methodological issue comes up that may sidetrack the discussion, ask the group how they want to handle it (usually it can be deferred and discussed with just the subset of learners who are interested in deeper methodology).

B. Keep the learners active.

1. Ask the learners to vote on what they would do clinically before the article is discussed. Ask them to write down their recommendations and pass in their scripts anonymously to avoid embarrassment.

2. When someone asks a question, NEVER ridicule them.

3. Turn questions back to the person asking or to the entire group: 'What does the group think?', 'Can anyone help out here?'

4. Call on people only when they feel comfortable and know it is 'OK' not to know.

5. Ask challenging (but not intimidating) open-ended questions: 'What do the authors mean by a randomized trial?' vs 'Is this a randomized trial?'

6. When bias might be present in an article, ask the group to decide if it might be important. If present, in what direction would it influence the results, i.e. would it widen or narrow a difference between groups? Do a worst case scenario analysis. Would this bias, if present and affecting all members of a group, reverse the analysis? (in other words, could this bias be a fatal flaw?)

7. When discussing diagnostic tests, go right to likelihood ratios (omit sensitivity, specificity, prevalence, etc.), go straight to the relevant 2×2 table and help the learners generate the appropriate proportions and calculations, asking them as you go along to express what the calculations mean in words. Only afterwards ask them to put names to these concepts, like sensitivity, specificity, etc.*

8. Summarize specific points during the session; check if it's OK to move on to the next topic. Stop from time to time to synthesize and summarize to show the group that there is a set of take-home messages even though full closure may not have occurred.

9. Time out: when particular problems or successes are occurring in the group dynamic, call 'time out' to divert attention to the group process rather than the clinical problem. Examine with the group what is occurring in the interaction, then call 'time in' to return to the clinical problem. Time outs can be especially useful when the teacher senses tension: call a time out, tell the group you sense tension and ask them what's going on.

C. Show your enthusiasm for critical appraisal in general and look for opportunities to compliment your specific set of learners and the work they are doing.

D. Novelty (once your team become adept at critical appraisal).

1. Use more controversial clinical topics and articles.

2. Use articles that come to different conclusions on the same topic.

3. In non-clinical situations, use 'role play' and scenarios. For role play, if people are reluctant, ask them to just play themselves, in the situations they find in their daily work life. Other situations to try include: courtrooms and malpractice claims, formal debates, point-counterpoint (appoint individuals to each role), hostile residents (or consultants!) on teaching rounds.

4. Introduce a 'quick challenge' for 'snap diagnosis': for an article with a fatal flaw, especially if you sense or discover that the group has not prepared in advance, start the session with: 'Quick, is there a fatal flaw in this paper and if so, what is it?'

Learning climate

A. Learners must feel comfortable identifying and addressing their limitations.

1. Be open about your own limitations and the things you don't know.

2. Use educational prescriptions (see page 33).

3. Periodically, make it a point to say that no one knows everything and that is why we are all here.

4. Encourage people to ask questions.

5. Have fun.

6. Provide feedback. Nod your head or make some reinforcing comment, especially when a correct response is given to a question or someone brings up an important issue.

B. Fight 'critical appraisal nihilism' ("No study is perfect, so what good is any of the literature?").

1. Select good articles, especially at the start.

2. Put the article into perspective in terms of what is known in the research area. This may be the first clinical trial of a new treatment.

3. Ask learners what they would look for in (or, if they are keen to do research, how they would design) a better study on this clinical issue.

4. Remind the learners that they have to use what is available in the literature for clinical decision making. Application of critical appraisal to clinical decision making is a positive process: not using critical appraisal can result in mindless adoption of faulty practices. Mindlessness is more nihilistic than questioning and seeking the right answer.

5. Separate innocent and possible problems from fatal flaws.

6. Help learners sort the literature and the clinical practice it supports into three categories: definitely useful, incompletely tested and definitely useless.

7. Remind the learners that it may be the editors' and not the authors' fault that insufficient information is provided in the published article.

* Credit for the original compilation of this list goes to Martha Gerrity and Valerie Lawrence

* Like lots of the elements of EBM, these concepts are not difficult but their jargon can be mystifying, so if you can orient students to the numbers and get them to say what they mean, you can later apply the usual terms, hopefully now demystified.

C. How to handle statistics.
1. Note the difference between statistical significance and clinical importance.
2. Use the 'statistics isn't important' technique. As a tutor, don't permit the session to turn into an attempt to teach statistics. Tell group members that study methods, samples, clinical measurements, follow-up and clinical conclusions are what's important and that statistics are merely tools to help these processes. If good methods were used, the investigators probably went to the effort to use good statistics (the 'trust 'em' mode). If bad methods were used, good statistics could never rescue the study (garbage in/garbage out; the frog is a frog and not a prince).
3. Suggest the quick and dirty sample size calculations such as the inverse rule of 3 on page 107.

Group control of the session

A. Discuss the goals of the session at its beginning and check along the way on whether it's making progress, especially if the discussion seems to be getting off track.

B. Learners' agenda versus teacher's agenda.
1. Try to go with the learners' agenda as much as possible. They will not learn all there is to know about critical appraisal in one session – remember how long it took you to learn it.
2. Let the group generate their own agenda for a specific session. This may lead into uncharted territory but learning will often be increased. The unlikely outcome is that closure may not be achieved, so be on guard to reassure (and, if you can't stand the chaos, provide direction).
3. Evaluate at the end to see if all goals were accomplished and how the next session could be more productive, more learner centered, more active, more stimulating and more fun.

C. When individuals try to dominate the discussion, put down others or 'know it all', take a 'time out' and ask the group to discuss individual responsibilities to the group. This should facilitate discussion of individual responsibilities and provide energy for individuals to take more responsibility (by the loud ones lightening up and the quiet ones contributing more).

D. When individuals or the whole group clam up and won't participate (not unusual at the first session).
1. Wait the 'magic 17 seconds'. No one can stand silence for more than about 5 seconds and the tutor who knows

(and believes!) this can outwait any group or member, no matter how long it takes. Refrain from jumping in to fill the silence yourself or they'll know that they don't have to take responsibility for their learning.
2. Take a 'time out' and ask the group members to discuss individual responsibilities to the group in terms of participation.
3. A possible script of questions to get a clinical problem + clinical article session going:
● How should we manage this clinical problem?
● What was there about the clinical article that supports that clinical decision (if unanimous) or those different decisions (if group members disagree on management)?
● (At this point it often becomes clear that some, and maybe all, group members haven't read the article). Does anybody need time to scan the article? (If so, you may want to give them 5 minutes to see what they can glean from it.) Alternatively, you could ask them to identify the features of an article that would be most helpful to them, then assign paragraphs of the methods section to pairs of learners and have them report back to the group on how well the article met their information needs.
● In the subsequent discussion, tease out and label the critical appraisal guides (emphasizing their generic importance rather than just how well they were met by the article).
● If the group is stalled, you could give them the guides, assigning one each to pairs of group members, have them work for a few minutes in pairs and report back to the group what they concluded and how it affects their clinical decision.
● What can we conclude and use in our clinical practice? Everyone agree?
● On which clinical issues did we achieve closure? On which not? See, lifelong learning is necessary!
4. Another question to foster discussion: The methods may be sound but are the results compelling? Concepts to bring out include statistical versus clinical significance, number needed to treat, etc.

E. Cures for the 'jumping around' or 'tangent' syndrome.
1. Remember that this syndrome is not always, or even usually, a disease. It regularly leads to long-lasting competencies in the areas under discussion, especially when the disparate elements are brought together by a skilled tutor.
2. Fill in the blank spaces on a blackboard (laid out with your mind's-eye framework of the relevant list of critical

appraisal guides) as the group comes up with and discusses the relevant issues. This will allow an unstructured discussion in which learners can generate criteria, points, etc. in any order that naturally arises, yet close with a coherent, ordered summary of the key guides and issues.
3. Check your watch frequently to see how the process is going. If a lot is being generated, don't worry about keeping a particular order or you'll risk stifling creativity and active learning.
4. Try to come up with 'segues' or transitional comments to tie what might appear to be tangential issues back into the clinical business at hand.

F. Capitalize on disagreements by asking for their bases in evidence or its critical appraisal. Where possible, reconcile them as arising from the application of different critical appraisal guides or from different interpretations of evidence related to the same guide. These reconciliations can be used to involve the rest of the group and to achieve closure on the particular issue.

G. When a learner asks a question directly to the tutor, allow the question to deflect onto another member of the tutorial, by pausing or by invitation. This can accomplish two things: (a) increase the group participation, and show them that they can teach each other, (b) buy time for you to think, in case the answer isn't immediately apparent to you but you don't want to admit that too soon!

Jargon
1. Explain a concept first, then label it with the jargon term. Better yet, get the group to explain the concept.
2. Ask learners who use jargon to explain the term to the rest of the group.

Finally
Remember that those learning to practice and teach EBM usually progress through two or three levels of expertise:
1. They become very good at sniffing out biases in articles (but don't yet know their consequences). They become highly critical and risk becoming entrenched nihilists.
2. They progress to being able to identify both the presence and direction of bias, so that they can sort out whether it's tending to produce false-positive or false-negative conclusions (and can be reassured when the latter makes a positive conclusion even more, rather than less, clinically relevant). They are ready for at least intuitive sensitivity analyses. You'd like your learners to get at least this far by the end of their training.

3. They progress further and suggest (or want to learn about) ways in which the study that produced the flawed evidence could have been designed or executed that would have prevented or overcome the bias. These learners may become interested in pursuing additional education in applied research methods and should be nurtured like other budding scientists (recognizing that their colleagues may not want to pursue these methodological discussions as part of the clinical discussions).

3. The main part of the journal club session is spent in a discussion critically appraising the evidence found in response to the clinical problem the club identified two sessions ago (we'll call it problem A) and about which it selected evidence for detailed study one session ago. The evidence is critically appraised for its validity and applicability and a decision made about whether and how it could be applied to future patients cared for by members of the journal club. This is the 'pay-off' part of the session and every effort should be made to ensure that 'closure' is reached. Ideally, a CAT is generated along the way, for discussion, revision and distribution to all the journal club members.

The actual order of these three parts of the journal club meeting could be reversed, depending on local preferences and tardiness!

Grand rounds and clinical conferences

Most hospitals hold weekly sessions in the auditorium for either their entire clinical staff or one of its departments. These sessions, which go by different names in different places, are conducted in order to discuss health issues of common interest and to try to accomplish continuing education and continuing professional development. They vary enormously in their subject matter (from molecular medicine to health reform) and in the passivity of their audience and in many hospitals patients have long since disappeared from the scene.

A common thread is the attempt to instruct the audience and transfer facts to them. Alas, as we learned back in the

Introduction, such instructional forms of CME, although they may increase knowledge, don't on average bring about either useful changes in clinical behavior or improvements in the quality of care.

Could a return to the grand round of a former era improve the situation? Building on that tradition and emphasizing some principles of EBM, these meetings could take on a different flavor and convert the audience from passive to active mode. The tactics are the following:

1. The rounds begin by focusing on a specific individual patient in the care of the presenters and the patient (whenever possible), images of the patient and undigested clinical data about the patient are presented.

2. The audience are required to assess this evidence, to generate opinions on its normalcy and diagnostic, prognostic or therapeutic implications and to report their individual opinions to the assembly by show of hands. To eliminate embarrassment and encourage participation, this reporting can be done anonymously by ticking diagnostic forms and then executing two or three exchanges among neighbors so that subsequent shows of hands are known not to represent the reporter's own opinion.* Of course, this solution is unnecessary in lecture halls equipped with anonymous, keypad voting systems.

3. A critical appraisal of the relevant evidence on the diagnostic, management or other issues raised by the case is presented in an interactive fashion, requiring the audience to offer opinions on its validity and applicability.

4. A hand-out is provided at the end of the round, summarizing both the relevant evidence and the critical appraisal guides for determining its validity and clinical applicability. In this fashion, an actively participating audience not only take stands on the appropriate evaluation and management of a real patient, but also receive a carry-away reinforcement

* It works! The author has used this approach over 100 times, with clinical audiences from five continents, and reckons that it produces participation rates of over 80%. A videotape of such a round (Clinical Disagreement about a Patient with Dysphagia) is available from the Centre for Evidence-Based Medicine in Oxford.

and set of guides that they can apply in other, similar situations.

Lectures (for preclinical students and clinicians of all ages and stages)

This entry may appear to be out of place! How could lectures, especially for preclinical students with no clinical skills or clinical judgment, focus in an active, interactive fashion on the care of individual patients? Well, they can, based on two realizations. First, even first year premedical students already have life experiences of a wide array of illnesses: all fear contracting AIDS, most have a relative with symptomatic coronary heart disease and many know someone with breast cancer. On the first day of school, they possess an array of personal clinical examples from which to consider the entire range of EBM topics. Second, there are unorthodox ways of employing lecture halls filled with students in ways that encourage active learning around EBM. This is perhaps best introduced by an example and the one that we will employ is a lecture to a first-year premedical class in biostatistics and epidemiology at Oxford.*

1. A clinical scenario is presented (on overheads), describing the clinical history and physical examination of a patient the speaker was called to see in an emergency room (in brief, a man who smells of alcohol and feces comes in complaining of a rapidly enlarging abdomen).

2. The students are asked to form pairs and write down the two most important facts they've been given about the patient and the two most likely explanations for his presentation. The lecturer then leaves the room for 5 minutes.

3. On return (to the sound of 60 active discussions!), the students report back their judgments and it quickly becomes apparent that there is remarkable preclinical consensus on what are considered 'clinical' issues of diagnosis.

* A videotape of this lecture (A Stercoraceous Man with a Swollen Abdomen) is available from the Centre for Evidence-Based Medicine in Oxford.

Table 4.6.3 A clinical scenario to initiate problem-based learning around an issue in therapy

You learn that a 54 y/o man with NIDDM (on oral hypoglycemics) whose myocardial infarction you treated 6 months ago has died suddenly at home. Wondering whether you could have done more for him, you review his notes and confirm that his was, in fact, a low-risk inferior MI with no complications whose blood sugar was elevated on admission (13 mmol/L) but settled down within 3 days.

In view of the success of 'tight control' of IDDM in preventing or postponing retinopathy and neuropathy, you wonder if a more aggressive treatment of his NIDDM might have postponed his untimely death. On the other hand, you well recall how one of your Profs back in medical school insisted that insulin was atherogenic and how you should back off insulin doses when diabetics developed angina pectoris.

So you form the clinical question: 'Among patients with NIDDM who are having MIs, does tight control of their blood sugar reduce their risk of dying?'

On your own or with help from the librarian at your local postgraduate center, you find the attached article: Malmberg K et al Randomized trial of insulin-glucose infusion followed by subcutaneous insulin treatment in diabetic patients with acute myocardial infarction (DIGAMI Study). J Am Coll Cardiol 1995; 26: 57–65.*

Read it (to possibly help you, we've included bits of a book on how to read clinical articles) and decide:
1. whether it answers your question;
2. if so, what the answer is;
whether you and your hospital colleagues should review how you are treating diabetic patients with myocardial infarctions.

---

* It can also be found on the disk version of *ACP Journal Club/Evidence-Based Medicine* or via MEDLINE using the terms: diabetes mellitus AND myocardial infarction AND publication type=randomized controlled trial.

4. The students are then asked to identify the next most useful bit of evidence about their diagnostic explanations and the ensuing discussion around the precision and accuracy of clinical signs and symptoms introduces sensitivity, specificity, pre- and post-test probabilities, likelihood ratios and the like for later use by the faculty teaching the rest of the course.

5. Once the diagnosis and initial treatment are discussed, the issue of long-term management arises and a journal article reporting a randomized trial is distributed. Students are asked to form quartets in order to take and defend stands on whether the treatment advocated in this report should be offered to the patient. The lecturer then leaves the room for 10 minutes.

6. On return (to the roar of 30 therapeutic debates!), the students again report back their judgments and why they've decided to accept or reject the therapeutic recommendations in the published paper. The discussion introduces another host of methodological topics around descriptive and inferential statistics, statistical significance, clinically useful measures of efficacy and other topics for later use by the faculty throughout the rest of the course.

The other teachers in this course kept coming back to this patient example as they introduced the principles and methods of epidemiology and biostatistics. The students reported (in addition to enjoyment) the growing realization of the manifest relevance of understanding some epidemiological and biostatistical methodology to their goals of becoming effective clinicians.

Workshops on how to practice EBM

Although clinical learners can and do acquire the skills and knowledge for practicing EBM 'on the job' as they proceed through their careers (and this is the only site where they learn how to integrate external evidence with individual clinical expertise and apply the synthesis to patients), many learners also seek opportunities for more concentrated and focused education in its critical appraisal components. For the last 15 years, such opportunities have been provided in

the form of workshops of a few hours' to a few days' duration. Originated at McMaster University in Canada, the workshop format has spread to other centers and countries and has been organized by various academic and professional groups, including a group of UK medical students who, impatient with the pace of change in undergraduate medical education, organized and ran their own 5-day workshop!* These workshops have four elements in common.

First, the learning is problem based and is typically centered around clinical scenarios describing actual patients who have been in the care of one of the faculty, accompanied by relevant research evidence (usually from the clinical literature), and calling for the learners to generate and answer questions about the clinical situation. Initially, the external evidence is provided, but later it may be the result of searches performed by the participants. By the end of the workshop, the participants will be expected to begin to pose their own questions about their own patients. An example of a clinical scenario with its citation appears in Table 4.6.3 and similar 'packages' are prepared for each of the disciplines (medicine, surgery, general practice, etc.), addressing issues in diagnosis, prognosis, therapy, systematic reviews, harm, economic analysis and quality of care.

Second, learning tends to occur in small groups of 5–10 participants with one or two tutors/facilitators who are skilled in teaching EBM and in running small groups. This provides an environment that encourages active learning and often replicates the clinical team settings in which EBM will be practiced subsequently. While carefully avoiding behavioral therapy, these groups also instruct and encourage their members in more effective and efficient team function by developing and following rules such as those that appear in Table 4.6.4. Each group meeting begins by setting an agenda for the session (including setting aside time for breaks, evaluation, future planning; agreeing on the clinical problem, the roles of group members, the edu-

* Named OCCAMS for Oxford Conference on Critical Appraisal for Medical Students and involving students from England, Scotland, Northern Ireland, Germany, Sweden and Croatia.

cational tasks and the evidence to be appraised; getting on with it (calling 'time out' when either the process or the content is getting bogged down); evaluating this session;

Table 4.6.4 How small groups succeed in learning EBM (or anything else)

1. By taking responsibility (individually and as a group) for showing up and on time; by learning each other's names, interests and objectives; by respecting each other; by contributing to, accepting and supporting individual and group rules of behavior, including confidentiality; by contributing to, accepting and supporting both the overall objectives of the group and the detailed plans and assignments for each session; by carrying out the agreed plans and assignments, including role playing; by listening (concentrating and analyzing, rather than simply preparing your own response to what's being said) and by talking (including consolidating and summarizing).

2. By monitoring and (by using time in/time out*) reinforcing positive and correcting negative elements of both:
- 'process', regarding educational methods (reinforcing positive contributions and teaching methods; proposing strategies for improving less effective ones) and responsibility (identifying behaviors, not motives; encouraging [e.g. with eye-contact, verbally] non-participants; quieting down [e.g. move them next to tutor] overparticipants); and
- 'content': unclear, uncertain or incorrect facts or critical appraisal principles/ strategies/ tactics.

3. By evaluating selves, each other, the group, the session and the program with candour and respect, 'celebrating' what went well (and should be preserved) and identifying what went poorly, focusing on strategies for correcting/ improving the situation.

* Time in for the teaching/learning portions of the session, especially when using role play, time out for discussions of effective/ineffective teaching/learning methods and group/individual behavior.

and planning for the next one. Thus, the learning focuses on the five steps that form the major chapters of this book:

1. forming answerable questions;
2. searching for the best evidence (workshops usually include individual tutorials by librarians experienced in teaching searching skills);
3. critically appraising the evidence (the major focus of most workshops);

4. integrating the appraisal with individual clinical expertise and applying it in practice (this element can only be carried out when workshops are spread out over longer periods of time, with regular clinical responsibilities taking place between sessions); and
5. self-evaluation.

Given the foregoing, the selection of participants (in addition to responding to consumer demand and general interest) seeks individuals who are already receptive to EBM (skeptics make important contributions to workshops and are welcome additions to the converted) and are likely to be able to apply what they learn in their clinical practice. Most evaluations suggest that small groups made up of clinicians in the same discipline (e.g. general practice, surgery, nursing, etc.) learn best, as they can work on scenarios specific to their disciplines and more readily see how they might apply the results of their growing skills in practice. The exceptions to this rule are methodologists such as epidemiologists and biostatisticians, who are often used to functioning in disparate groups and can contribute to one of any make-up. The play of chance and small numbers (surgical specialities often are underrepresented) sometimes makes for unusual combinations of disciplines and these often require additional attention to be sure that alternative scenarios are presented to maintain relevance for all members.

Third, lots of time is set aside for small group meetings, individual study and meetings of ad hoc interest groups. Educational materials are sent out well in advance (with a reassurance that not all have to be mastered before the workshop!). A typical schedule is shown in Table 4.6.5. Tutors meet daily to report progress, to make mid-course corrections in the workshop and to identify and solve problems in group function and learning (their training occurs in the 'how to teach EBM' workshops described in Chapter 5). Plenary sessions are kept to a minimum and deal only with issues best communicated in a lecture or lecture-audience participation format (a review of EBM, how to pose answerable questions, an introduction to information searching, etc.) and a final feedback and evaluation session where par-

Table 4.6.5 A typical schedule for a workshop on how to practice EBM

Time	Sunday	Monday	Tuesday	Wednesday	Thursday	Friday
0800		Tutors meetings				
0900		Plenary sessions on forming questions, searching, etc.				Small groups
1000		Small groups	Small groups	Small groups	Small groups	Small groups
1100						Evaluation
1200		Lunch				Good-bye
1300		Individual study or ad hoc interest group meetings or individual searching				
1400	Tutors' meeting					
1500						
1600	Small groups	Small groups	Small groups	Small groups	Small groups	
1700	Small groups	Small groups	Small groups	Small groups	Small groups	
1800	Supper					
Evening	Social	Study	Social	Study	Social	

ticipants hand in their evaluation forms and suggest improvements for future workshops.

Some workshops are held in one-day or half-day sessions, spread out over longer periods of time. Less efficient for organizers, these often merge with the journal clubs described above and provide more opportunities for integrating the critical appraisals with individual clinical expertise as the EBM skills are acquired.

Fourth, participants and organizers keep in touch after the workshops in order to continue to trade ideas on how to practice EBM, how to improve future workshops and so that some of the participants can move to the next level of not only practicing EBM but teaching it as well. These workshops will be described in Chapter 5.

Further information

Get on the WWW and browse the educational resources of the Centre for Evidence-Based Medicine in Oxford by contacting the Uniform Resource Locator: http://cebm.jr2.ox.ac.uk/

Individuals interested in attending or organizing workshops in how to practise EBM can contact either the Department of Clinical Epidemiology and Biostatistics at McMaster University (1200 Main Street West, Hamilton, Ontario, Canada L8N 3Z5) or any of the Centres for Evidence-Based Practice in the UK (for example: http://cebm.jr2.ox.ac.uk/ will get you to the Website for the Centre for Evidence-Based Medicine in Oxford).

The educational materials for each session include:

1 A clinical scenario, based on a real patient we've seen on our service.

2 The clinical question that arose from caring for this patient.

3 The searching strategy we employed in looking for external evidence.

4 The results of that search.

5 A description of the skills–training elements of Part B of the session.

6 A blank worksheet of users' guides for critically appraising that evidence for its validity and potential clinical usefulness.

7 A completed worksheet, showing what we thought of it – the answers might not be right, but they're ours! This is for the benefit of those who are teaching the course and for evaluation purposes so they can be separated from the pre-circulated materials and saved for later.

8 A CAT summarising the article. Again, these can be separated from the pre-circulated materials.

If you aren't an old hand at teaching EBM, you might want to attend one of the *Workshops on how to teach EBM* that are held at various locations each year. These workshops include plenty of chances to develop and perfect your skills in leading sessions on the critical appraisal of articles from the clinical literature. They also explore the evidence sources that are used in this course. To find out when and where the next Workshop is being held, look on our web page: http://cebm.jr2.ox.ac.uk/

Several of the teaching methods that can be used in this course are described on pages 188–97 of *Evidence-based Medicine: how to practice and teach EBM*, by D Sackett, W Richardson, W Rosenberg, and R Haynes (published by Churchill-Livingstone).

There are several different ways to lead the discussions of the clinical scenarios and papers in these sessions:

1 We suggest that you begin all of them by being sure that the learners understand the patient's biological and clinical problem and the 3- (or 4-) part clinical question.

2 The ultimate objective is to help learners apply the users' guides to the paper and understand them well enough to be able to apply them to subsequent papers. You can accomplish this in different ways:
   – you could ask them (either altogether or in groups of two to four) to apply each of the guides in turn, and discuss them and their application in sequence. This approach is more efficient but less self-directed, and is useful when time is scarce or the group is reticent about expressing their views.
   – at the other extreme, you could initiate a free-form discussion by asking learners to take and defend their stands on whether they would apply the paper's conclusions to the patient, and then draw the guides out of this discussion. This approach encourages self-directed learning, but is less efficient than the tutor-directed approach and requires a group who are comfortable expressing their views.

3 We urge you to end each session by evaluating it with the learners, identifying ways that they, you and the readings could be improved for next time.

The other resources that we called upon in running this course were:

1 Two of our local librarians – Anne Lusher and Robin Snowball – who ran the session on MEDLINE searching and have developed a teaching package for undergraduate and graduate learners. They are members of the Centre and can be contacted through us if you want additional information on how they conduct their sessions.

2 Reference to the book and cards inside it – these pages are colour-coded to match the relevant cards. *Evidence-based Medicine: how to practice and teach EBM*, by D Sackett, W Richardson, W Rosenberg, and R Haynes (published by Churchill-Livingstone in 1997 for £14.99).* You may already have another reference with which you're more familiar or find more useful.

3 For you and your learners to make optimal use of this syllabus you and they will need easy access to computers that include both CD-ROM and Internet access.

4 *Best Evidence*, a CD with cumulated abstracts and other materials from *ACP Journal Club* and *Evidence-based Medicine*, two journals of critically appraised articles from an array of clinical journals covering internal medicine, general practice, obstetrics and gynaecology, paediatrics, psychiatry, and surgery. This resource can be ordered from the BMJ Publishing Group (PO Box 295, London WC1H 9TE; Tel: 0171 387 4499 and ask for Subscriptions; Fax: 0171 383 6662; e-mail: bmjsubs@dial.pipex.com).

5 One of the MEDLINE searching systems (we used *WinSPIRS*). MEDLINE can now be searched on the Internet: http://www3.ncbi.nlm.nih.gov/PubMed/

6 CATMaker, a software programme we developed for analysing, summarising and storing critical appraisals. It can be obtained from our Centre and from our website.

7 Our website (**http://cebm.jr2.ox.ac.uk/**) where we keep several banks of clinically useful measures on the precision and accuracy of clinical exam and lab test results (SpPins, SnNouts, sensitivities, specificities, likelihood ratios), on the power of prognostic factors, and on therapy (NNTs, RRRs and the like).

8 For demonstrating *Best Evidence*, MEDLINE searching, and the CATMaker we used a computer projector device that displayed the contents of a computer screen onto the wall for all to see.

This program (and other similar programs that we have developed) have been used in rounds for medical students, house officers, registrars and consultants. Thus, we have confirmed (to ourselves at least!) that this approach can be used by clinicians at any age or stage in their careers.

* Copies are available at a 20% discount when purchased in large numbers for a workshop. Contact Louise Ashworth at Churchill-Livingstone (0171 282 8303).

If you are interested, similar manuals have been developed for use by general physicians in primary care, mental health and paediatrics.

We look forward to receiving feedback and suggestions for how we might improve this course.

Sharon Straus
David Sackett

Centre for Evidence-based Medicine at Oxford

This session on therapy provides two options:

1 A patient with hypertension and the SHEP study to discuss the use of diuretics for decreasing the risk of stroke, **or**

2 A patient who is having a comprehensive geriatric assessment and an article about geriatric assessment for decreasing dependency and nursing home admission.

The SHEP study is more challenging providing issues around validity and applicability to discuss.

The geriatric assessment paper is less challenging but of interest to people who may be involved with planning geriatric services.

Complete sets of handouts are provided for each patient scenario.

Critical appraisal of a clinical article about therapy (suggested minimum time allotment: 60 minutes)

EBM SESSION

1

TUTOR'S GUIDE

Therapy and asking answerable clinical questions

Learning objectives

1 To introduce the concept of critical appraisal and the use of critical appraisal guides and worksheets.

2 To learn how to critically appraise evidence about therapy for its validity, importance and usefulness.

3 To introduce the number needed to treat (NNT) as a clinically useful measure that can be derived from research reports.

4 To stress the application of research evidence to the individual patient.

There are several different ways to lead the discussion of this and the subsequent four sessions (and they are discussed in greater detail on pp188–97 of *Evidence-based Medicine*):

1 We suggest that you begin all of them by being sure that the learners understand the patient's biological and clinical problem and the 3- (or 4-) part clinical question.

2 The ultimate objective is to help learners apply the users' guides to the paper and understand them well enough to be able to apply them to subsequent papers. You can accomplish this in different ways:
   – you could ask them (either altogether or in groups of two to four) to apply each of the guides in turn, and discuss them and their application in sequence. This approach is more efficient but less self-directed, and is useful when time is scarce or the group is reticent about expressing their views.
   – you could initiate a free-form discussion by asking learners to take and defend their stands on whether they would apply the paper's conclusions to the patient, and then draw the guides out of this discussion. This approach encourages self-directed learning, but is less efficient than the tutor-directed approach and requires a group who are comfortable expressing their views.

3 We urge you to end each session by evaluating it with the learners, identifying ways that they, you and the readings could be improved for next time.

4 Ideally, our scenario should begin with trying to identify a systematic review that can answer our clinical question. Systematic reviews may be more difficult to appraise and so we've included them in Session 5. However, you may want to consider tackling systematic reviews first.

B Asking answerable clinical questions (suggested minimum time allotment: 30 minutes)

Learning objectives

1 To learn why the formulation of 3- (or 4-) part questions about our patients is necessary:
   - for identifying educational tasks that can be accomplished in limited time
   - for focusing searches for evidence.

2 To learn how to generate 3- (or 4-) part answerable clinical questions from our patients.

Asking answerable questions is discussed in detail in Chapter 1 of *Evidence-based Medicine*.

The strategy we suggest that you follow is aimed at illustrating the importance, strategies and tactics of formulating clinical questions, especially through paying attention to 3- (or 4-) parts of the question.

After a brief introduction, you could break the learners up into groups of two and ask them to discuss patients they've cared for in the previous week. You could then challenge them to generate questions they think are important concerning their patients' therapy, diagnosis, prognosis. Then you could reconvene the larger group and get some of them to volunteer their questions so that you can, as a group, review and refine them until you agree that they ought to be answerable.

We urge you to keep track of these questions for use in later sessions devoted to searching for the best evidence (especially if you already know that there is good evidence about them). The feedback we've received is that your learners will be disappointed if you simply forget the products of this session and fail to use them in later searching sessions.

PART A

Critical appraisal of a clinical article about diagnosis (suggested minimum time allotment: 60 minutes)

Learning objectives

1 To learn how to critically appraise evidence about diagnosis for its validity, importance and usefulness.

2 To introduce:
   - the concept of pre-test probability and its derivation from clinical expertise
   - the concepts and calculation of sensitivity and specificity (minor emphasis)
   - the concept and calculation of likelihood ratios (major emphasis)
   - the concept and calculation (or simpler derivation from the nomogram) of post-test probability from the pre-test probability and the likelihood ratio as a clinically useful measure that can be derived from research reports.

3 To understand the superiority of likelihood ratios over sensitivity and specificity.

4 To stress the application of research evidence about diagnosis to the individual patient.

PART B Searching the evidence-based journals (suggested minimum time allotment: 30 minutes)

Learning objective

1 **To learn how to search the evidence-based journals of secondary publication (Note: tutors will need to decide whether to start teaching clinicians how to find the best evidence as we've begun here, with the easiest sources of high-yield, high-quality evidence (but employing searching systems that incorporate 'fuzzy logic' and take away the challenge of being highly precise in specifying search terms). The alternative (preferred by some tutors of EBM) is to start at the other extreme (which we introduce in Session 4) with the low-yield, variable-quality primary literature which requires much stricter specification of the clinical question and the employment of search terms drawn from methodological as well as clinical considerations. Subsequent sessions cover sources of evidence (the Internet and the Cochrane Library) that call for intermediate searching skills.)**

Searching the electronic versions of the evidence-based journals is so much easier (no need to know anything about database structures, MEDLINE MeSH terms etc.) and so much more rewarding (only the 2% of articles that are methodologically sound as well as relevant get into it) that more and more of us start learners off with this source rather than any of the MEDLINE systems.

The contents of the ACP Journal Club and *Evidence-based Medicine* are available on CD, as *Best Evidence*. (It can be ordered from the BMJ Publishing Group, PO Box 299, London WC1H 9TD; Tel: 0171 387 4499 (subscriptions); Fax: 0171 383 6662; e-mail: bmjsubs@dial.pipex.com.)

You could use this resource for finding evidence about some of the questions your learners generated last week (you may want to try out a few of them prior to the session so that you are sure to have some 'winners').

We've included a summary sheet on the different sources of evidence and their properties.

We also suggest that you start the members of the group thinking about their own questions for their presentations in Sessions 6 and 7. The following page is a reminder that you might want to distribute.

- Take one of your patients who presented an important problem in therapy, diagnosis, prognosis or harm.

- Formulate that problem into a three-part question (the patient, the manoeuvre and the outcome), based on what you learn from Session 2.

- Do a search for the best evidence based on what you learn from Sessions 3–5 (lots of help available from us or the library team).

- Critically appraise that evidence for its validity, importance and usefulness.

- Integrate that appraisal with clinical expertise and summarise it (in a one-pager if you wish).

- Present it to the rest of us at one of the final sessions. (Certificates will be given to presenters.)

Your turn: case-presentations

EBM SESSION

TUTOR'S GUIDE

**Prognosis
and
introduction
to the
CATMaker
software**

PART A
Critical appraisal of a clinical article about prognosis (suggested minimum allotment time: 60 minutes)

Learning objectives:

1 To learn how to critically appraise evidence about prognosis for its validity, importance and usefulness.

2 To introduce:
– the concept of inception cohorts and their importance in the validity of studies of prognosis
– the concept (but not the tedious calculation) of precision and confidence intervals.

3 To stress the application of research evidence about prognosis to the individual patient.

PART B
Introduction to the CATMaker (optional) (suggested minimum allotment time: 30 minutes)

Learning objective

1 To become able to use the CATMaker.

In this part of the session, you can show the learners how to use the CATMaker to generate their own one page summaries of published trials. The advantages of the CATMaker include its ability to calculate for them the clinically useful measures of the effects of therapy and their confidence intervals.

Obviously, in order to demonstrate it, either you or a co-tutor has to know how to drive this beast, and tuition on how to run it is part of our workshop on *How to Teach EBM*.

It would be useful to have a partially-developed kitten that you could load for your demonstration. You could create one yourself or use the one that comes with the CATMaker – this is a diabetic with hyperglycaemia at the time of a myocardial infarction, and summarises the DIGAMI randomised trial of tight control. To learn how to obtain copies of the CATMaker, see our web page: http://cebm.jr2.ox.ac.uk/

At the close of this session, you could encourage the learners to start searching on potential topics for their presentations in Sessions 6 and 7.

PART A Critical appraisal of evidence about harm (suggested minimum time allotment: 60 minutes)

Learning objectives

1 To learn how to critically appraise evidence about harm for its validity, importance and usefulness.

2 To introduce the concepts (but not the tedious calculations) of some clinically useful measures of harm:
   – the NNH (number of patients one needs to treat in order to harm one of them)
   – relative risk (RR) and the odds ratio (OR).

3 To stress the application of research evidence about harm to the individual patient.

PART B Searching the primary literature (suggested minimum allotment time: 30 minutes)

Learning objectives

1 To understand how clinicians can use the efforts of the US National Library of Medicine to classify and catalogue original articles.

2 To understand how to construct high-quality searches of the primary literature using:
   – medical subject headings (MeSH)
   – 'limiters'
   – words from the free text
   – methodological filters.

3 To be introduced to other databases of primary literature.

We've never seriously considered trying to teach this skill without the collaboration of expert colleagues from the library. We strongly encourage advance planning with local librarians, trying out searches on the questions generated by your learners in earlier sessions, so that you can show them some tangible, useful results, easily and quickly obtained (rather than going in cold and producing a long, slow, complicated and ultimately fruitless search that will turn them all off).

One note of caution: many librarians are used to working with researchers rather than clinicians, and they are understandably concerned that searches get **all** relevant citations. The needs and wants of clinicians are very different, and are usually met by **just one or a few** citations of high methodological standard and relevance. We urge you to discuss this with your librarian colleagues before you start this session.

Efficient EBM searching strategies developed by the research librarians in the Health Information Research Unit at McMaster (that trade off the sensitivity and specificity of your searches) are included with this package.

If your learners haven't done their searches for their presentations in Sessions 6 and 7, the last few minutes of this session would be a good time to demonstrate some previously sorted out successful ones, plus some 'problem' searches.

Systematic reviews and searching the Cochrane Library

PART A Critical appraisal of a systematic review (suggested minimum time allotment: 60 minutes)

Learning objectives

1 To learn how to critically appraise evidence from a systematic review for its validity, importance and usefulness.

2 To introduce the concept that overview is superior both to individual trials (because of greater precision and the rejection/confirmation of clinically important subgroups) and to traditional review (because of greater validity).

3 To stress the application of research evidence about prognosis to the individual patient.

PART B Searching the Cochrane Library

Learning objectives

1 To learn how to look for evidence in the Cochrane Library, including:
– Cochrane reviews
– DARE (the Database of Abstracts of Reviews of Effectiveness)
– the clinical trials registry.

2 To gain information about the Cochrane Collaboration (and encouragement to join it!)

In demonstrating the Cochrane Library, you might want to have done enough homework to have identified some systematic reviews that are of great relevance to your learners.

Presentations and surfing the Net

PART A **Presentations**

Depending on the number of learners who are presenting their own cases, you may find that you require just one session for these (and for the introduction to the Cochrane Library). In that case, you can either shorten the course to six sessions or give them one 'open' session in which they can come to you for advice and help with searching for, critically appraising and summarising their evidence or to raise other issues in critical appraisal, EBM etc.

PART B **Surfing the Net**

Learning objective

1   To learn how to search for evidence on the worldwide web

In this part of the session, learners can be shown how to access the web including, if you wish, the web page for the NHS R&D Centre for Evidence-based Medicine in Oxford (http://cebm.jr2.ox.ac.uk/) where there are data banks of clinically useful measures on the precision and accuracy of clinical exam and lab test results (SpPins, SnNouts, sensitivities, specificities, likelihood ratios), on the power of prognostic factors, and on therapy (NNTs, RRRs etc.), including entries from the articles used in this syllabus, plus the CATMaker and links to several other centres and sources of evidence. The handout may help orient them to the web.

PART A Presentations

The other half of the participants will present their patients, questions, critically appraised topics and clinical conclusions.

PART B Feedback and celebration

Learning objectives

1 To evaluate the course ('Evaluation of practising EBM')
   - to improve it for the next time you give it
   - to provide feedback to the developers of this course back in Oxford.

2 To permit the learners to evaluate their own performance ('Am I practising EBM?').

3 To decide where you and the learners want to go from here in continuing to learn and practice EBM (e.g. clinical rounds, academic half-days, journal clubs, etc. which are described on pp 185–206 of *Evidence-based Medicine*).

The final portion of the session can be spent evaluating the course. The attached forms permit written feedback, and a discussion will be held on general issues.

We urge you to devote special attention to discussing and deciding what to do with what has been learned and how to continue to improve and use this set of clinical, EBM and self-directed learning skills on clinical rounds, in academia half-days, journal clubs etc.